Ending the Food Fight

ENDING the FOOD FIGHT

Guide Your Child to a Healthy Weight
in a Fast Food / Fake Food World

David S. Ludwig, M.D., Ph.D.

Director, Optimal Weight for Life Program
Children's Hospital Boston

with

Suzanne Rostler, M.S., R.D.

HOUGHTON MIFFLIN COMPANY

BOSTON • NEW YORK

2007

To my parents, MIRIAM and VICTOR,
who have devoted their lives to
the fight for social justice

———

And to DAWN

For information about permission to reproduce selections from
this book, write to Permissions, Houghton Mifflin Company,
215 Park Avenue South, New York, New York 10003.

Visit our Web site: www.houghtonmifflinbooks.com.

Library of Congress Cataloging-in-Publication Data
Ludwig, David, date.
Ending the food fight : guide your child to a
healthy weight in a fast food/fake food world /
David S. Ludwig with Suzanne Rostler.
p.   cm.
Includes bibliographical references.
ISBN-13: 978-0-618-68326-0
ISBN-10: 0-618-68326-7
1. Obesity in children—Popular works.
2. Weight loss. I. Rostler, Suzanne. II. Title.
RJ399.C6L83 2007
618.92'398—dc22   2006030465

Printed in the United States of America

Book design by Victoria Hartman

MP 10 9 8 7 6 5 4 3 2 1

CONTENTS

NOTE TO READER

All of the stories in this book are real, representing the actual experiences of Optimal Weight for Life (OWL) Program patients, parents, and staff. Only minor changes have been made to maintain confidentiality or for editorial purposes. One story, Jared in chapter 2, includes material from several patients to demonstrate the range of issues that can arise in a medical evaluation.

ACKNOWLEDGMENTS

This book was written by hundreds of people, including patients, colleagues, friends, and mentors. It has been my great privilege to translate their words to you.

First, I would like to express my gratitude to Suzanne Rostler, who seemed to float out of the sky, like Mary Poppins, when the project was in need of help. A huge thank-you to Mollie Katzen for convincing me to write this book and helping the project take shape. I am also grateful to Alison Rose Levy and Susan Gilbert, who helped develop the foundation for this work.

A warm thanks to Chris Swett for developing the recipes with me. After countless hours by phone, I can't wait to meet you in person next time I'm in Berkeley. Natalie Engler provided creative assistance, and Juliana Weinstein helped with research.

I am grateful to Linda Loewenthal of the David Black Literary Agency for her abiding friendship and professionalism. Thanks also to my editor, Jane Rosenman (you are a delight), and the creative team at Houghton Mifflin.

Many colleagues provided invaluable consultation, advice, and critical review of the manuscript, including Susan Albers, Jennie Brand-Miller, Bill Dietz, Len Epstein, Michael Jacobson, Allison Lauretti, Marlene Schwartz, Barry Sears, Kelly Sinclair, Melinda Sothern, Walter Willett, and Sandy Woodruff.

A special acknowledgment to Joe Majzoub, my career mentor. There are no words to express the depth of gratitude I feel for your wise council these past fifteen years. I am also grateful to Jeff Flier, in whose lab I learned the fundamentals of obesity research.

My gratitude to family, friends, and spiritual mentors who have, directly or indirectly, supported this project: Ben Brown, Amy Fox, Julian Gorodsky, Thich Nhat Hanh, Sant Keshavadas, Michael Linfield, Peter Ludwig, Victor and Miriam Ludwig, Rick Malley, Patrick McCarty, Shanti Rubenstone, Hale Sofia Schatz, Alison Shaw (if you're ever near Arlington, Massachusetts, and want the best therapeutic massage of your life, look her up), and Lino Stanchich. Heartfelt appreciation to Dawn Pallavi, for inspiration and support throughout this past year (check out her culinary institute, The Natural Epicurean, for the best whole foods cooking classes in Austin, Texas).

I am deeply grateful to the members of my research group for exploring the mysteries of science with me and for their patience and understanding as I wrote this book. Cara Ebbeling deserves special recognition: for the past seven years, she has led or assisted in most of our studies, helped formulate hypotheses, written grants and manuscripts, and supervised others. Also Michael Agus, Tracy Antonelli, Cristin Aubin, Diego Botero, Kamryn Eddy, Sheila Ellenbogen, Preethi Fonseka, Hope Forbes, Erica Garcia-Lago, Michael Leidig, Lenny Lesser, Margaret Lovesky, Gina Masse, Beth Monroe, Dorota Pawlak, Mark Pereira, Niki Philippas, Marta Ramon-Krauel, Kaitlin Rawluk, Erinn Rhodes, Sandy Salsberg, Kelly Scribner, Linda Seger-Shippee, Kelly Sinclair, Janet Washington, and Lindsey Wong.

Of course, this book wouldn't have been possible without the Optimal Weight for Life (OWL) Program staff, dating back to 1996. OWL staff not otherwise mentioned above include Michelle Chagnon, Jennifer Crossland, Roseann Cutroni, Linda Daley-O'Brien, Amy Fleishman, Bob Flynn, Anat Hampel, Jan Hangen, Alison Hoppin, Inger Hustrulid, Ana Jiminian, Colleen Kochman, Roberta Laredo, Carine Lenders, Karen Lewis, Maryanne Lewis, Nicole Marcus, Bob Markowitz, Cathy Noonan, Voula Osganian, Mary Jane Ott, Laurie Raezer, Brian Ramos, Hans Ritschard, Shahna Rogosin, Johanna Sagarin, Nina Sand, Tamyka Sanford, Lilly Santiago, Rochelle Shubin, Leslie Spieth, and Kina Thomas.

Finally, I wish to express my gratitude to the thousands of OWL patients and families who have taught us all so much.

Brookline, Massachusetts
August 2006

INTRODUCTION

During my pediatrics residency training in the early 1990s, I helped care for Grace, a three-year-old girl who was admitted to the hospital with failure to thrive. This condition — usually caused by a chronic medical problem, improper nutrition, or neglect — results in poor weight gain and stunted growth. However, Grace's condition was unusual: she had gained no weight at all in nine months, but her growth had continued at an entirely normal rate. In addition, her appearance was striking, especially compared to photos taken of her in infancy. Over the previous year, all of her normal baby fat had melted away, yet her muscles were remarkably preserved, making her look like a tiny bodybuilder.

After a few days of fruitless investigation, we finally discovered that Grace had a rare abnormality in a region of the brain called the hypothalamus, which controls body weight. Somehow her brain was sending her body the message to shed every single ounce of fat. But since she was otherwise healthy, the growth of other body tissues continued uninterrupted. Unfortunately, the surgery needed to treat Grace's condition produced damage to the part of the brain that controls satiety, the sensation of fullness we get after eating. Almost immediately after recovering from surgery, Grace developed a ravenous appetite and a significant problem with overeating. Through the next few years, Grace gained a great deal of weight, going from being substantially underweight to seriously overweight. Grace's mother, with support from our medical team, struggled to control her daughter's hunger and slow down her weight gain.

By the end of my pediatrics training, the obesity epidemic in the United States was in full swing. Influenced in part by my experience with Grace, I decided to pursue a career in obesity and joined a basic research laboratory studying the biological factors that affect body weight. I became fascinated by the beauty and complexity of the body's weight-regulating systems. Under most circumstances, these systems help maintain a near-perfect balance between calorie intake and calorie expenditure. Without these systems, our weight would fluctuate wildly, as did Grace's. Just the calories in an extra bagel and cream cheese each day could cause a thirty-five-pound weight gain in one year.

During my five years in basic research, I helped discover a gene that can make laboratory mice fat and might contribute to human obesity. However, I came to believe that the discovery of new genes was unlikely to provide a cure for obesity anytime soon. After all, our genes haven't changed much in the past thirty years, but rates of obesity have more than doubled. So in 1996, I left the basic laboratory, began researching new dietary approaches to obesity in people, and developed the Optimal Weight for Life (OWL) Program at Children's Hospital Boston. Since then, OWL has grown from a staff of two to one of the largest clinics for overweight children and their families in the country.

When people find out what kind of work I do, they often say something like, "You treat overweight children? That must be so sad." Sometimes I do feel sad. Overweight people, and especially children, are subject to incessant teasing, abuse, and discrimination. The stories of our patients can at times be heartbreaking. And sometimes I feel angry. Soft drink companies spend millions of dollars on advertising targeting children, but OWL has to fight with insurance companies for only a few hundred dollars to cover the treatment of an obese child. More often I feel joy. In addition to the small, day-to-day victories that you'll read about throughout this book, there are great triumphs. For instance, in chapter 2 you'll meet Michael, who came to OWL at age fourteen. At that time, he was 5 feet 4 inches tall and weighed 220 pounds; he had high cholesterol, high triglycerides, fatty liver, and insulin resistance. Now nineteen years old and 5 feet 10 inches tall, Michael has reached an optimal weight of 155 pounds, and all of his obesity-related complications have resolved.

If you are the parent of an overweight child, or if you want to prevent a problem from developing in the future, this book is for you. In the following pages, I'll share with you what we've learned from fifteen years of research and from working with thousands of families just like yours. I'll introduce you to OWL patients who have made dramatic breakthroughs and others who are still struggling. And I'll walk with you, step by step, as you and your family take this journey to health.

PART I

A View from
the Battlefront

OVERWEIGHT AND OVERPOWERED

Wherever we went, there was food, and wherever there was food, we had a fight," said Bobby's mother, Amanda. Bobby had developed a serious weight problem by age fourteen, and Amanda was terribly concerned about his health.

"We dreaded going out for dinner," she said. "Bobby would try to place an order directly with the waitress, always for the biggest thing on the menu, so I had to be the food police. At first I'd give him some leeway, but he kept pushing and pushing for more. He'd get belligerent, like we were starving him. Then I'd lose my patience and get angry."

At parties, Amanda would "cringe" when her son helped himself to large portions of food. "I'd see other people watching him and knew what they were thinking: What's wrong with these people? How can they let their kid be so heavy and eat that way?"

Dinner at home was no better. Bobby would try to serve himself from the counter. Amanda would tell him to sit down, that she'd get his food. "Then I'd eat quickly, so I could run interference if he got up for seconds," she said. But his two lean siblings were allowed to have

seconds, so Bobby felt there was a double standard. "You don't understand," he'd say. "I am hungry. Besides, it's my business; let me do
what I want. I don't know why you even care!" Eventually, Bobby's
father would lose his patience. "That kid's going to eat himself to
death!" he'd yell. Although Amanda tried to keep the peace, on most
nights everyone left the dinner table in a huff. "It felt like a battleground," she remarked.

AND SO IT IS for millions of families in America today, fighting a
war that takes place on three fronts.

The first battle is *within the child*. It's the battle that erupts whenever your child is hungry, pitting mind against metabolism. His body
tells him to eat, but his mind says no. Summoning willpower, he vows
to resist temptation. But his body sends stronger, more urgent signals
to supply the calories needed to survive. Outflanked, his mind has no
choice but to succumb. By this time, he is ravenous and ready to grab a
bag of potato chips, a sugary drink, or whatever other high-calorie
product is nearby. These unwholesome foods will fill him up for a
short while, but the struggle within will begin anew the next time
hunger strikes.

The second battle takes place *in the family*. Desperate to help, you
find yourself monitoring and restricting what your child eats. You may
criticize him for eating too much or too often, or for choosing the
wrong foods. You get angry with yourself for being so critical. It's just
that you're concerned about your child's weight and fearful that his
health will suffer because of it. Despite good intentions, you and your
spouse argue over what to do, perhaps even blame each other. Siblings
tease him about his weight and complain because you no longer keep
certain foods in the home. Instead of providing respite from the day's
stress, the home becomes another front where the food fight is waged.

The third battle takes place *around us*. It's the conflict between
families like yours that want to support their children's health and an
environment that undermines your every move: the commercials for
soft drinks and fast food targeting our kids; the junk food sold in

schools; the supermarket shelves bursting with sugary cereals, candy, and chips. These "foods," if we can call them that, are everywhere and taste good — a seductive combination for children.

Yet your child needn't be seduced. To end the food fight, children need an eating and activity plan that works with their basic biology, promoting weight loss without causing deprivation. And parents need age-appropriate strategies to help their children develop healthful habits without causing conflict. I ask families to consider the forces that have led so many children to gain so much weight. Their bodies invaded by junk food, their minds tricked by endless advertisements, our kids have become collateral damage in a world that places private profit over public health. This knowledge may make people angry, but anger can be powerful medicine.

Today, Bobby is winning his food fight. After eighteen months in OWL, his body mass index has decreased by four units, equal to about twenty-five pounds. He has discovered the importance of a healthy diet and developed strategies to avoid eating out of anger or boredom. Just as important, the family has learned to work together. Whereas Amanda used to keep junk food in the house exclusively for Bobby's siblings, the rules have changed. All family members have equal access to all foods at home, and only healthy foods are allowed in the house. That means if Bobby's siblings want junk food, they have to eat it someplace else. His father has become more patient and lets Bobby play a more active role in decision making. Despite the occasional argument, "things at mealtime are definitely more peaceful now," Bobby said. But for millions of other families, the war rages on.

The Scope of the Problem

Maintaining a normal weight has never been harder than it is today. In the United States, the percentage of overweight children ages six to eleven has doubled in the past twenty-five years, and the percentage of overweight teenagers has tripled. One out of three children — a staggering 30 million kids — is too heavy. Forget the stereotypes about childhood obesity affecting mainly the urban and rural poor. It is a problem that touches all racial and ethnic groups, all geographic areas of the country, and all socioeconomic levels. My patients are white, black, Hispanic, Asian, and Native American, with roots all over the world. They come from some of the poorest neighborhoods and some of the wealthiest. They come from families where Mom is a home-maker and families where Mom is a surgeon.

Never before has there been a generation in which so many kids are so heavy so early in life. This crisis facing our kids mirrors the epidemic of overweight and obesity in adults, except that the stakes are much higher. The consequences for children will be vastly greater because they will be carrying more weight for much longer, and also because this burden is occurring during critical stages of childhood growth and development.

Pediatricians now regularly diagnose obesity-related conditions in children that used to strike only middle-aged and elderly adults, such as high blood pressure, high cholesterol, fatty liver, and sleep apnea. Just fifteen years ago, we virtually never saw children with type 2 diabetes, a potentially life-threatening disease caused primarily by obesity. Today this condition, previously called adult-onset diabetes, affects children as young as eight years old.

Just as being overweight jeopardizes the physical health of children, it also can be devastating to their emotional well-being and social functioning. One study found that when fifth- and sixth-grade students were shown drawings of children with various physical conditions — one who was obese, one in a wheelchair, one with crutches, and so on — and asked whom they would like to have as a friend, they picked the obese child last. Other research shows that being very overweight in childhood impairs a person's quality of life as severely as having cancer.

What will happen to overweight kids as they grow older? Studies show that when overweight adolescents reach adulthood, they are less likely to have finished school, less likely to be married, and more likely to be living in poverty. Children who develop type 2 diabetes face the devastating prospect of heart attack, kidney failure, amputation, and other life-threatening complications before they turn thirty. Shockingly, overweight adolescent girls have almost a threefold increased risk of dying by middle age compared to lean girls, even after taking into account other lifestyle factors that could affect health. And according to a study we did with Jay Olshansky at the University of Chicago, life expectancy may decline in the United States by up to five years in the next few decades, roughly equal to the impact of all cancers combined, as a direct result of the childhood obesity epidemic.

Don't I Just Have Fat Genes?

Why can some children eat whatever they want and remain thin, whereas others try hard to eat right but gain too much weight? Genes, those tiny parts of our DNA that determine the color of our eyes and hair, also affect body weight.

Some scientists have proposed a theory for the obesity epidemic that humans possess: "thrifty genes." Historically, these genes (also called "fat genes" or "hungry genes") helped humans gain extra weight when food was plentiful so that they could survive during times of scarcity. According to this theory, thrifty genes were favored by evolution and passed down through the generations. But now, in an environment of abundance, these genes drive people to become and remain obese.

Although genetic factors clearly influence an individual's predisposition to be heavy, there are two important problems with this theory. First, there have been long periods in history during which humans have lived amid abundance without gaining excess weight. Since the end of World War II, for example, most Americans, Europeans, and Japanese have had plenty to eat, but obesity rates didn't start climbing until the 1970s in America, the 1980s in Europe, and the 1990s in Japan.

The second problem with the thrifty gene theory is that the biological forces governing our weight work in both directions: some promote weight gain, others weight loss. While being too lean would have been a problem for our ancestors, so would being too fat. Obese women, for instance, have high rates of infertility and complications during pregnancy — very unfavorable traits from an evolutionary standpoint. An obese hunter-gatherer also would have been most attractive to — and least able to escape from — the local saber-toothed tiger. Thus, from an evolutionary perspective, excess weight isn't always an advantage.

Biologically, our bodies have evolved control systems to maintain weight in a remarkably stable range, sometimes termed the *body weight set point*. If food intake drops too low, hunger will urge us to eat more to regain the missing calories. Just try fasting for a day and see how you feel. But other systems push in the opposite direction. After a huge Thanksgiving dinner, for example, most of us want nothing to do with food for a while and have a smaller appetite the next day.

Like genes, the environment can push our inner weight control systems in one direction or the other. Let's suppose a group of obese Americans — eating fast food, drinking sugary beverages, and not getting enough physical activity — were magically transported to rural Japanese villages in 1960. What would happen as they began to eat a more healthful diet and do more manual labor? They'd start losing weight, and the weight would probably keep coming off for several years. If local scientists observed this transition, they might wonder whether people from the United States had a "spendthrift gene," making it hard for them to hold on to weight. Similarly, if American children today were transported back in time to America in the 1960s, most childhood obesity would disappear.

Research from our laboratory suggests that we don't need a time machine to readjust our body weight set point. Changing the types of foods we eat can produce fundamental changes in metabolism that make losing weight much easier, as we'll discuss in chapter 3.

The take-home message is this: Genes aren't destiny, especially when it comes to body weight. People with an inherited predisposition aren't doomed to a lifetime struggle with obesity. There have always been a few overweight children, but the dramatic increase in childhood obesity over the past three decades is without precedent. Our genes haven't changed very much during this time. What has changed is the environment in which we live — a "toxic environment," according to Kelly Brownell of Yale University.

The Toxic Environment

To see just how toxic our environment has become, let's take ourselves out of it for a moment and pretend that we're part of a fact-finding team sent to a disaster area to survey the wreckage and piece together what happened. The disaster, in this case, is the epidemic of childhood obesity.

Our mission begins in the kitchen of the modern American home. We see cabinets stocked with processed foods and snacks; vegetable bins with room to spare; household garbage cans filled with fast food wrappers, pizza cartons, and soda cans. We see parents racing home after long hours at work, stressed-out and drained of energy. It's too late to cook dinner, so they stop along the way for a carryout meal or take the family out for fast food. The portions of these meals are enormous; the soda cups are the size of water jugs. Once occasional treats, fast food, sweets, and soda have become regular fare.

Our next stop is the school. In the hallway, we see vending machines that sell soda, candy, and chips. In the classroom, we see first and second graders learning to do arithmetic with books that feature M&M's and other junk food. Cash-strapped schools have franchised the cafeteria to fast food companies and reduced or eliminated physical education classes and afterschool recreation opportunities.

Now we return to the home, where children spend many hours a day watching TV. A typical child sees ten thousand food commercials each year, mainly for fast food, sugary breakfast cereals, and other high-calorie, low-quality snack foods. Kids sit for hours playing video and computer games. Teenagers seem to live at the computer. Entire days pass when they don't move around enough to work up a sweat.

Then we take a look outside. Many poor neighborhoods have no parks or playgrounds where children can run and play. The prospects for outdoor activity aren't much better in many upscale neighborhoods. Many suburbs are built without sidewalks, making it dangerous for children to walk or ride their bicycles to school.

Our team's conclusion? The physical and social landscape in America today seems ideally designed to make children fat.

FAKE FOOD

❖ Nutritionally speaking, our kids have gotten in with the wrong crowd. Instead of eating foods that nourish them and help them maintain a healthy weight, they have befriended "fake food." These foods are nutrient-poor and pack on the pounds. If they were people, we wouldn't invite them into our homes or drive our children to play dates with them. We'd encourage our children to make real friends. But right now, many of us load up our kitchen cupboards with foods made in factories and drive our children to fast food restaurants.

Fake food — highly processed products bearing no resemblance to anything found in nature — fuels the battle between mind and metabolism. It is loaded with calories but devoid of real nourishment. It fills us up briefly but depletes us of the vitamins, minerals, and other key nutrients our bodies need. Containing artificial flavors that mask its true tastelessness, fake food provides a momentary feeling of pleasure that quickly passes. Instead of satisfying our needs, it actually induces cravings and promotes overeating in our bodies' desperate attempt to replenish those missing nutrients.

Personal Responsibility or Social Responsibility?

Some people argue that it's unfair to blame the childhood obesity epidemic on an overabundance of fast food and fake food. The issue, they say, comes down to personal responsibility: parents are free to choose healthier foods and to teach their children to do the same. This is what the food industry wants us to believe. But in reality the situation is far more complicated. Expecting parents to exercise true freedom of choice in today's toxic environment is like expecting someone being swept up in a tsunami to swim away. Regardless of how hard we try, we are overwhelmed by forces beyond our control.

One of these powerful forces is a food industry that puts profit over pounds, corporate wealth over our children's well-being. Food companies pay advertising executives top salaries to convince children to consume the highest-calorie, lowest-quality products imaginable. Studies clearly show that kids are more apt to nag their parents for the foods they see advertised on TV and less likely to eat unadvertised foods. And when was the last time you saw an ad for broccoli, zucchini, or cauliflower?

We could resist the insidious influence of advertising were it not for two realities of modern life. One is that these foods are everywhere: convenience stores, supermarkets, highway rest stops, playgrounds, and friends' homes. Even so-called safe havens such as schools offer no refuge. It's just so easy, so convenient, so *normal* to choose fake food. Besides, many of them taste pretty good.

Biologically, humans are born with an innate preference for sugar, fat, and salt, nutrients necessary for infant growth. As children grow, their preferences normally broaden to include the complex range of tastes found in nature. If this were not the case, children long ago would have starved to death once they stopped breastfeeding.

Food manufacturers exploit our survival mechanisms by deliberately making their products extra-sweet, extra-fatty, or extra-salty, adding artificial flavor enhancers to make us crave them even more.

Food companies incessantly advertise these products to children during a stage of life when they are highly susceptible to manipulation. The result is that taste preferences become arrested in an "infantilized" state of development.

Patients of mine who emigrated from rural parts of China, Haiti, or other areas relatively free of advertising have told me that they initially experienced fast food as repulsive. But to children on a steady diet of fake food, chemically manipulated flavor becomes the norm. Eventually, an apple doesn't taste sweet, and vegetables seem completely inedible. And so our children get hooked on calorie-dense, nutrient-poor junk, fueling the battle between mind and metabolism that causes weight gain.

Supersize portions make the problem worse. With typical fast food meals weighing in at a full day's energy requirements, children lose the ability to regulate their food intake. Research shows that young children tend to eat the same amount at a meal regardless of whether they're given smaller or larger portions. Older children do much less well at balancing food intake with energy needs. Factors besides hunger, including how much food they are served, prompt them to overeat. These findings suggest that young children are in touch with the inner "satiety" cues that tell them when they are full, but older kids either lose these cues or their ability to recognize and respond to them. Supersizing may actually erode children's ability to know the difference between eating enough and eating too much.

The second reality of modern life that makes us so vulnerable to the influences of advertising is that we've stopped cooking. Our generation eats away from home more often than any other in human history. In the past, most food that children consumed was prepared by people who knew and loved them. Now we have delegated this fundamental responsibility to strangers whose primary consideration is profit, not our health. The nutritional wisdom passed down through generations from time immemorial has been interrupted; our intimate connection with food is being lost. To end the food fight, we must reconnect with the foods that nourished our grandparents and their grandparents.

Ending the Food Fight

Like many parents we see for the first time in the OWL Program, you probably feel overwhelmed by how difficult it is to help your child lose weight. You may have begun to pack your child's lunch instead of relying on cafeteria food, or you may have convinced other parents to join you in offering only wholesome snacks during play dates. And you may have encouraged your child to be more physically active. But no matter what supports you put in place, powerful and unforeseen forces threaten to sabotage your every step.

I've illustrated this situation in Figure 1.1. The toxic environment overwhelms our weight control systems (biology) and undermines our willpower (psychology), making it almost impossible to eat well and stay physically active (behavior). As a result, children gain excess weight, sparking conflict at home.

However, these forces are not all-powerful. During my ten years as director of the OWL Program, I have witnessed hundreds of families join together to end the battle against their bodies and against each other. As shown in Figure 1.2, your family can become a protective shield against the toxic environment. Fun physical activities replace TV viewing. Fake food no longer fills your pantry; instead, you stock your shelves with wholesome foods that can be easily prepared and packed for lunches and snacks. You may not eat together as a family every night, but dinners are now planned and prepared on a schedule. Instead of a battleground in which the food fight is waged, the home becomes a place of peace.

But let's not stop here. Having made peace at home, your family can join together with other families, as shown in Figure 1.3. You can reach out into the community to help clean up the toxic environment,

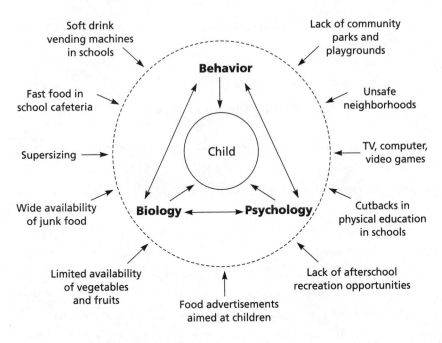

Figure 1.1 Child Vulnerable to the Toxic Environment

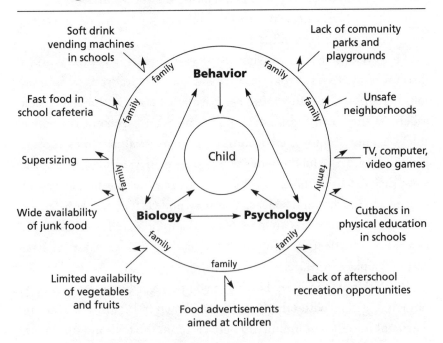

Figure 1.2 Child Protected from the Toxic Environment

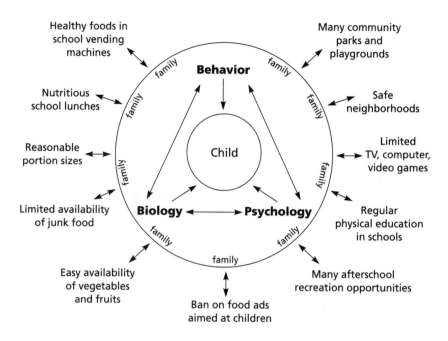

Healthy foods in school vending machines

Nutritious school lunches

Reasonable portion sizes

Limited availability of junk food

Easy availability of vegetables and fruits

Ban on food ads aimed at children

Many community parks and playgrounds

Safe neighborhoods

Limited TV, computer, video games

Regular physical education in schools

Many afterschool recreation opportunities

Behavior

Child

Biology ←→ **Psychology**

family

Figure 1.3 Families Joining Forces to Detoxify the Environment

working with your schools and communicating with elected officials to bring about sensible policy changes that can reduce childhood obesity. Vending machines that once offered soda and candy bars are filled with nourishing foods. Afterschool recreation programs provide fun, safe opportunities for physical activity. And fast food restaurants as we know them today close for lack of business, replaced by restaurants serving nutritious meals. Ultimately, we all benefit. With the foundations in place to support our children's health, we can lay down our arms as the food fight ends.

So let's get started . . .

WELCOMING CHILDREN
TO WEIGHT LOSS:
A Day at the OWL Clinic

Eight ten A.M., my office in the Optimal Weight for Life clinic.

Jared, fifteen years old, and his mother, Beth, arrive. Although it's a hot summer day, Jared is wearing a baggy sweatshirt with the hood pulled up, covering part of his face. He sinks into a chair, shoulders slumped, and pulls a Game Boy from his pocket. His mother sighs. She tells him to put the game away, take off his hood, and pay attention.

Jared scowls. He puts down the Game Boy and stares at his shoes.

"How are you today?" I ask. Silence.

"Answer the doctor," Beth says to her son.

"Fine," says Jared, without making eye contact.

I try another tack. I ask them both, "Whose idea was it to come today?"

Jared, without saying a word, slowly raises a finger and points it at his mother.

I ask Beth why she decided to bring Jared to OWL. She tells me that Jared has always been on the heavy side, but over the past few years, his weight has shot off the growth chart. At the last visit to his pediatrician, they learned that Jared has high cholesterol and border-line high blood pressure. "The doctor said Jared could get diabetes," Beth says. "And I'm worried that he always seems sad. His teachers have told me he gets teased a lot about his appearance and he doesn't have many friends."

"Jared," I ask, "are you concerned about your appearance or your health?"

"No," he says.

"Yes he is," Beth insists. "There are days that he comes home from school crying, and he's been refusing to undress for gym in the boys' locker room."

Jared glares at his mother and fumes in flat-out adolescent rebellion. Beth looks exasperated. It's an armed standoff.

"So you're not thrilled about being here today?" I ask Jared.

"She forced me to come," he says. I consider this response a small victory; at least he answered in a complete sentence.

Sometimes children come to my office ready and willing to deal with their weight. Jared is more typical, having been brought to the clinic at the urging of his doctor, seemingly against his wishes. But what he isn't saying is that of course he's concerned about his weight. He's terribly concerned. How could he not be in a society as weight obsessed as ours? What's more, he and his mother essentially want the same thing: for Jared to be healthy and feel good about himself. The tragedy is that so much of their energy has gone into conflict that there's very little left to deal with the weight problem.

Some children have serious underlying psychological problems, such as depression, that require specialized attention. And some families struggle with major stresses, such as alcoholism, that call for professional counseling. In most cases, however, simple, straightforward behavioral techniques can begin to defuse these conflicts right away, often leading to profound changes in family dynamics.

It's time for a peace treaty. I ask Beth whether I have her permission to make an unusual proposal. She says she's willing to try anything, since nothing has worked for them in the past.

"Jared, here's my proposition: No one will make you come to another appointment at OWL against your wishes. But since you're here today, I ask that you keep an open mind, participate in the conversation, and consider whether the OWL Program might have something to offer you." I look at Beth. She hesitates for a moment and then nods in agreement. Jared mumbles, "OK," and the mood in the room begins to lighten.

I would not use this approach with young children. Prior to adolescence, kids need clear limits from their parents. But for many teenagers to admit they have a weight problem, let alone take action to deal with it, empowerment is essential. Adolescence is a time of growing independence, self-assertion, and differentiation from parents. Teenagers need to feel acknowledged for who they are. They also need the freedom to make some of their own decisions and the space to deal with the consequences. Only then can they begin to take control of their behavior, redirecting their energies from rebellion to responsible action.

Having obtained Jared's temporary cooperation, I begin my clinical evaluation by looking for any underlying medical causes of his excessive weight gain and for possible complications that can result from his being overweight.

"Do you have problems with low energy or poor strength?" I ask. "What about great sensitivity to cold? Any changes in your skin or hair? Constipation?" These conditions provide clues to the presence of a hormone problem involving the thyroid, adrenal glands, or pituitary. Jared answers no to these questions.

"Do you have excessive thirst or frequent urination?" — signs of diabetes. Jared shakes his head.

"Any shortness of breath when you exercise or difficulty keeping up with other kids in sports?" I ask. Jared laughs self-consciously. "Every fat kid has that," he says.

"How about pains in your muscles, bones, or joints?" Jared admits that he does suffer knee and foot pain, especially when he's physically active, a common complaint among patients in our program. "Imagine walking around all day with a backpack loaded with your school-books," I say. "Now imagine how you'd feel if you could never take it off. Your body would soon start to get sore. That's what's happening to your legs."

The combination of shortness of breath and musculoskeletal pain during exercise can make it difficult for an overweight child to partici-pate in sports and active play, or simply to climb a flight of stairs. Un-able to burn off excess calories, he gains even more weight, making physical activity that much more difficult. Often the only way out of this vicious cycle is weight loss.

I ask about heartburn and indigestion. Jared says that about twice a week, he has a burning sensation in his chest after eating. "That's likely to be a condition called gastroesophageal reflux," I say, "and it can be caused or made worse by being heavy."

I continue with the medical evaluation, asking about loud snoring, difficulty breathing at night, and fatigue during the day. These can in-dicate a respiratory disorder known as sleep apnea, in which a person stops breathing for fifteen seconds or more dozens or even hundreds of times each night. Sleep apnea can be life threatening and require the use of a machine to help with breathing during sleep. This condition can place the body under great stress, producing changes in hormones and metabolism that lead to more weight gain. But once sleep apnea is diagnosed and adequately treated, weight loss often begins, sometimes almost effortlessly. And with weight loss, sleep apnea generally im-proves or resolves.

"Other medical problems?" I ask. "Any medications?" Steroids such as cortisone and some drugs used for psychiatric illness are known to cause weight gain. One medical issue, asthma, can be of particular concern in overweight children. Excessive body weight can cause wheezing by putting pressure on the lungs and restricting breathing. In addition, fat tissue releases substances into the blood-stream that cause airway inflammation and constriction, the hallmarks of asthma. The mainstay of asthma treatment is steroids, which leads to weight gain. And with continuing weight gain, asthma may worsen

— another vicious cycle that at times can be broken only by weight loss. Besides problems related to his weight, Jared has been otherwise healthy and is not taking any medication.

I then ask Jared, "Have you started to go through puberty yet?"

He looks at the floor. "Sort of," he says.

"His voice is just beginning to change," says Beth, concerned that puberty is getting off to a late start. Indeed, Jared does look young for his age. Beth thinks his "baby face," which lacks any sign of hair, is causing some of the teasing Jared experiences at school.

Many overweight children begin puberty early because hormonal changes associated with excess body weight can overstimulate the ovaries, testicles, and adrenal glands. In fact, the average age that girls have their first menstrual period has continued to decline during the past three decades in the United States, probably because of the increasing prevalence of childhood obesity. I routinely see overweight girls whose breasts have begun to develop by age eight and who have begun to menstruate by age ten.

Although overweight boys also tend to go through puberty early, some, like Jared, progress more slowly. A likely explanation for this is that fat tissue converts the male hormone testosterone into the female hormone estrogen. High estrogen interferes with the normal tempo of puberty and stimulates the growth of breast tissue in boys, a condition called gynecomastia.

Puberty can be challenging at any age, but children who experience it before or after most of their friends may face additional social pressures and emotional problems. An eight-year-old girl with breast development may look like a teenager and be treated in a way that is not appropriate for a child of her age. This can lead to confusion, shame, or precocious sexual behavior. Overweight boys who develop late and have gynecomastia can be subject to ridicule from peers, compounding feelings of embarrassment and leading to social isolation.

I ask Beth if there is a history of any medical problems in the family. Beth says that both she and Jared's father have always struggled with their weight. Beth's brother, who is also overweight, was recently prescribed a medication for high blood pressure. She pauses, then adds that her father recently suffered a stroke as a result of diabetes. Although genes are not destiny, family history provides insight into a child's risks for future diseases, I explain.

Then I broach a delicate topic. "Do you ever eat until you're really stuffed? Do you sometimes feel out of control when you eat? Have you ever tried to lose weight by not eating or by throwing up?" Answers to these questions can provide clues to a potential eating disorder. Although eating disorders are far more common among girls, they can happen in boys as well. Eating disorders such as bulimia nervosa (self-induced vomiting to lose weight) require urgent, specialized treatment that must take precedence over weight loss. Indeed, focusing on weight loss without first attending to underlying psychiatric problems can often make matters worse.

Major eating disorders are relatively infrequent among my patients, but many overweight adolescents engage in dysfunctional eating patterns such as binging, stealing food, and secretive eating. These behaviors can cause considerable shame, as well as conflict with parents.

Jared says that he has never tried to lose weight, let alone by making himself throw up. But he feels uncomfortably full after dinner some nights. Beth says that she has noticed food missing over the past few months. At first she questioned her memory, but then she began to find candy wrappers stuffed in the back of Jared's desk and in his pockets, and she knew something was going on.

I take a quick emotional read of the situation and decide it's time to dive in. "I'd like to ask about your eating habits," I say to Jared. "Would you say your appetite is small, medium, or large?"

"Medium," Jared says.

"Enormous," Beth says.

Giving an accurate diet history can be a challenge for anyone. Try for a moment to remember everything you ate yesterday, the day before that, a week ago. Most of us tend to underestimate the amount of food we eat and selectively remember healthy foods more than unhealthy ones. Studies have shown that obese individuals underestimate food intake to an even greater extent than lean individuals. For obvious reasons, it's difficult to obtain a meaningful diet history from a self-conscious, overweight adolescent. So for this part of the interview, I do my best to create a supportive and nonjudgmental atmosphere.

"Do we have your permission for Jared to be completely honest about his eating habits?" I ask Beth. "Can you guarantee that there'll be no negative consequences for anything he might reveal?"

"Absolutely," Beth says.

Playfully, I declare, "Nothing you say right now can or will be used against you in a court of law."

Evidently reassured, Jared proceeds to describe what I call SAD — the standard adolescent diet. On most mornings, he rolls out of bed at the last possible minute, then races off to the bus stop without having breakfast (yes, it is the most important meal of the day). At midmorning, he has a twenty-ounce fruit drink, the kind with 5 percent fruit juice — meaning 95 percent sugar water. His lunch in the school cafeteria is a fast food nightmare: chicken fingers, French fries, chocolate milk, cake, and another sugary drink. From the time he arrives at a friend's house after school until the time he goes to bed, he consumes a dizzying array of popcorn, chips, cookies, ice cream, and candy. On the two or three nights each week that he has a sit-down dinner with his family, he eats chicken or meat and potatoes or pasta, but he leaves the green vegetable on this plate untouched. All told, he has fast food most days of the week and consumes on average one liter of sugary soda every day. Research from our laboratory found that for every additional serving of soft drink per day, a middle school child's risk of becoming obese increased by a remarkable 60 percent.

Although the quality of Jared's diet is exceedingly poor, it's the rule, not the exception, for teenagers today. Most of the foods he eats are high glycemic (see chapter 3), high in energy density (calories per bite), low in fiber, low in nutrients, and low in satiety (how long a food keeps us full). As a result, he consumes hundreds of calories beyond his needs on a daily basis.

I thank Jared for being so honest about his diet. Then I ask him to tell me the difference between real food and fake food. He looks at me quizzically. "Simply put," I say, "real food comes from nature, fake food from a factory." I show him his diet record and ask him to consider each of the items he described and to circle each fake food. "Wow!" he exclaims after complying with this request. "I guess I'm eating a lot of the fake stuff."

Next I ask about Jared's lifestyle. "How physically active are you?"

"I throw a football around with friends after school," he reports.

"He's a couch potato," Beth says.

How many hours do you spend watching TV and playing video games?

"About two or three hours a day," Jared answers.

"At least five hours a day during the week and more on the weekend," Beth insists.

"Jared," I ask, "would you say that you spend at least thirty hours each week watching TV?"

"Yeah, I guess so. Almost a full-time job," he quips.

I say that I hope he is being well paid for all that TV viewing, considering how much trouble it's going to cause him. Research has clearly linked TV viewing to excess body weight in childhood and to increased risks for obesity and heart disease in adulthood (see chapter 4).

Now it's time for Jared's physical examination. His blood pressure is 136/80, on the high side for an adult, let alone for a teenager. His general appearance is normal, without any characteristic features of genetic syndromes that cause excessive weight gain. Although Jared is very overweight, the excess fat tissue is evenly distributed on his body, not located primarily around the midsection, and he has good muscle mass. These findings provide reassurance that he doesn't have an underlying hormone problem.

His skin has scattered stretch marks on the abdomen and thighs, common among overweight children and adults. Of greater concern are patches of dark, velvety skin around the nape of the neck. I point out this skin condition to Jared and Beth and ask whether they've ever seen this before. "I've been after him to wash more thoroughly," Beth says.

I scrub the affected area with an alcohol pad to demonstrate that the discoloration isn't dirt and won't come off. "It's a skin condition called acanthosis nigricans, indicating that insulin levels in the body are already elevated — a risk factor for diabetes." Noting Beth's anxious look, I emphasize that I have no reason to think Jared has diabetes now. With weight loss, the diabetes risk will subside, and the skin condition will fade.

Next I examine his eyes and vision and find no evidence of a brain disorder. The thyroid gland, located at the base of the neck, is entirely normal. Lungs, heart, and abdomen also are normal.

I ask Jared to undress fully and request that Beth leave the room. Jared appears hesitant. I explain that this is a normal and important part of a complete physical examination. When Jared finally takes off his shirt and shorts, I immediately understand his reluctance: he has a considerable amount of breast development, and his penis is almost completely buried in the fat around the pelvic area. I tell him that these conditions are common among overweight teenage boys and that there's absolutely nothing wrong with him. Once he loses weight and continues through puberty, the breast tissue will probably disappear, and his "private parts" will look just like those of other boys his age. Jared looks relieved.

He gets dressed. I call Beth back into the room, and we review the results of the blood test from earlier in the morning. The thyroid test is normal. Many parents, convinced that their child's weight gain is caused by a "slow metabolism," suspect hypothyroidism, although in my experience this is rarely the case. Jared's blood sugar is in the normal range, which means that he does not presently have diabetes. However, an additional test identifies insulin resistance, a major risk factor for the development of diabetes. His triglycerides (the amount of fat in the blood) are distinctly elevated, and his HDL (good) cholesterol is low; both are major risk factors for heart disease. In addition, a liver test indicates the possible presence of fatty liver, a potentially serious condition that can cause liver damage and even cirrhosis. Fortunately, all of these abnormalities improve with a good diet, physical activity, and weight loss.

Having completed the medical interview, exam, and laboratory analysis, I proceed with my assessment of Jared's weight problem. First, I call their attention to the growth chart. Jared is 5 feet 6 inches tall, just about average for a fifteen-year-old boy. Since he hasn't yet had his growth spurt, which occurs later in puberty for boys, I expect Jared to be tall, perhaps 6 feet. He seems pleased to hear this prediction. However his weight, at 205 pounds, is clearly out of proportion to his height.

I then calculate Jared's body mass index (BMI), a measure of body weight relative to height. For adults, a BMI of 18 to 25 is normal, 25 to 30 overweight, and over 30 obese. For children, BMI normally changes as they grow and develop, so BMI percentiles for age and gender are increasingly being used to classify weight status. Throughout childhood and adolescence, a BMI between the 3rd and 85th percentiles is considered to be normal, a BMI between the 85th and 95th percentiles raises concern for overweight, and a BMI greater than the 95th percentile indicates a serious weight problem (see Figure 2.1). Jared's BMI is 33, placing him well above the 97th percentile for his age and gender. Although Jared and Beth aren't surprised by this information, many families are shocked to find out just how serious the problem is.

I tell Jared I have good news and bad news. The good news is that there is no evidence of any underlying medical or genetic problems that might be contributing to his weight. Such problems tend to cause poor growth, delayed puberty (Jared is on the late side but still within the normal range for boys), low energy, low muscle mass, and other physical signs and symptoms. Fortunately, these problems occur in less than 1 percent of all overweight children.

The bad news is that there is no simple pill that will make his weight problem magically disappear.

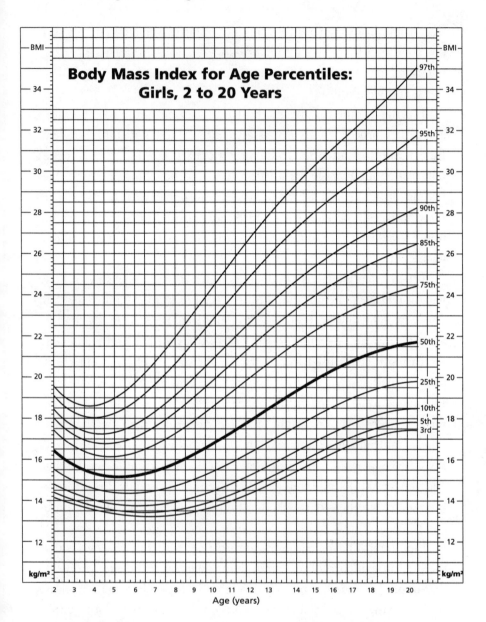

Figure 2.1 Determining Your Child's BMI Percentile

Using a calculator, find out your child's BMI as follows: Take weight (in pounds) and divide by height (in inches), divide a second time by height (in inches), and multiply by 703. Now refer to the proper chart, depending on your child's gender. Locate age along the bottom of the

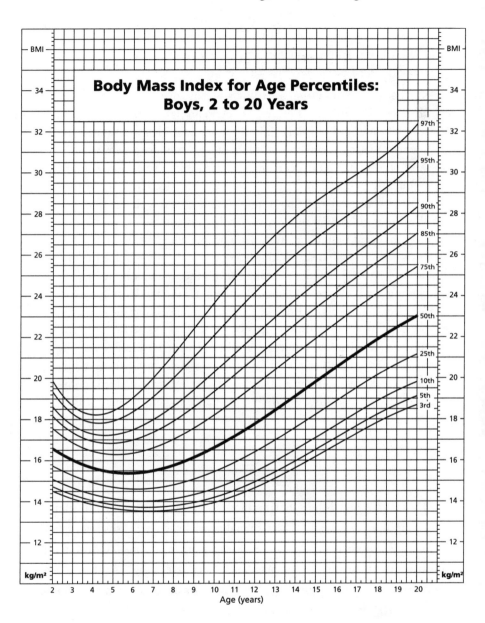

Body Mass Index for Age Percentiles: Boys, 2 to 20 Years

chart, then follow the nearest vertical line upward until you find your child's BMI; place a mark on that spot. The curving lines, with numbers ranging from 3 to 97 at the right, indicate your child's BMI percentile. In most situations, BMI percentile provides a good indication of body fatness. However, some individuals, such as bodybuilders, can have a high BMI with normal (or even low) body fat.

CAN YOU "CATCH" OBESITY?

❖ That was the question asked by a recent cover story in the *New York Times Magazine*. Researchers at Pennington Biomedical Research Center in Louisiana and colleagues have identified a strain of adenovirus that seems to cause laboratory animals to gain weight. And in a human study, evidence of past infection was found more frequently in obese compared to lean individuals. However, before we don biological agent body suits, let's keep a few things in mind. We don't yet know if this virus actually causes obesity in humans or is an innocent bystander. And many people who have been exposed to the virus remain lean. With further research, it is possible that infectious agents may join the long list of other biological factors, including many dozens of genes, that increase the tendency for some people to gain weight. But like genetic influences, specific cures for possible infectious causes of obesity are unlikely to be found in the foreseeable future. So a nutritious diet and an active lifestyle remain the best approach to prevent and treat a weight problem. In addition, good nutrition and physical activity have benefits for the immune system, possibly improving resistance to getting that virus in the first place.

I then give Jared the sobering facts about obesity and health. Being overweight at any age increases a person's risks for heart disease, type 2 diabetes, some forms of cancer, and many other serious conditions. In addition to these long-term problems, very overweight children and teenagers can suffer from a great number of immediate, and in some cases life-threatening, medical problems (see Figure 2.2).

Of particular concern, I tell Jared, is type 2 diabetes in childhood. When I did my training in pediatric endocrinology in the early 1990s, just about the only kind of diabetes we saw in children was juvenile-onset, or type 1, diabetes. Type 1 diabetes is an autoimmune disease unrelated to body weight in which the insulin-producing cells in the

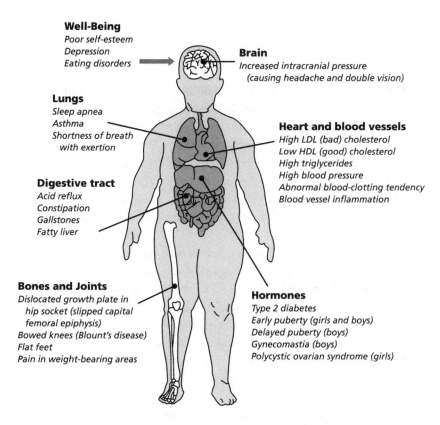

Well-Being
Poor self-esteem
Depression
Eating disorders

Brain
Increased intracranial pressure
(causing headache and double vision)

Lungs
Sleep apnea
Asthma
Shortness of breath
with exertion

Heart and blood vessels
High LDL (bad) cholesterol
Low HDL (good) cholesterol
High triglycerides
High blood pressure
Abnormal blood-clotting tendency
Blood vessel inflammation

Digestive tract
Acid reflux
Constipation
Gallstones
Fatty liver

Bones and Joints
Dislocated growth plate in
hip socket (slipped capital
femoral epiphysis)
Bowed knees (Blount's disease)
Flat feet
Pain in weight-bearing areas

Hormones
Type 2 diabetes
Early puberty (girls and boys)
Delayed puberty (boys)
Gynecomastia (boys)
Polycystic ovarian syndrome (girls)

Figure 2.2 The Complications of Childhood Obesity
Modified from Ebbeling et al., *Lancet* (2002), 360:473–82 (with permission).

pancreas are destroyed. Type 2, or adult-onset, diabetes, the kind strongly linked to excessive body weight and insulin resistance, used to occur only in adults.

"It's one thing for an obese forty-five-year-old to develop type 2 diabetes by age fifty-five and suffer complications at age sixty-five," I say to Jared. "It's quite another thing for an overweight fifteen-year-old to develop diabetes in his early twenties and have a heart attack in his thirties."

Jared starts to speak, but Beth cuts him off, bringing the conversation back to diabetes and its complications. Turning to me, she says almost plaintively, "I've been trying, time after time, to tell him about

JUDY'S STORY

❖ By the time Judy started preschool, her weight had begun to affect her self-esteem, according to her mother, Gloria. "She was the largest in the class, and the other kids started calling her names," Gloria said. "After school, Judy would come home upset, asking why she was heavier than everyone else." Gloria herself has had a lifelong struggle with weight and was the subject of teasing and taunts as a child. She didn't want the same thing to happen to her daughter. She was also concerned because obesity and diabetes run in her family.

The biggest challenge at home was that Judy absolutely hated vegetables. "It was always a struggle," Gloria recalled. "She'd take one look at the vegetables on her dinner plate and say, 'Gross! I'm not eating that,' without even taking a bite. I'd tell her, 'You're not leaving the table until you've tried it.' So she'd forced down a bite, sobbing, sometimes choking herself in the process. I'd feel awful that it had gotten to that point. Then my husband would get involved, and it was downhill from there. These quarrels were emotionally exhausting for everyone — it was ripping my heart out."

Another challenge was Judy's sedentary lifestyle. With both parents working demanding jobs, finding the time to encourage physical activity was difficult. "We'd get home from a long day, tired, and fight with each other about who would go for a walk with Judy," Gloria said. Once they got outside, Judy "would whine that the walk was too long."

Gloria brought Judy to OWL at age six and a half years. During her first visit, we devised a behavioral plan using some of the methods discussed in chapter 6. To defuse tension at dinner, we asked Gloria not to pressure her daughter to eat vegetables and not even to mention the word "vegetables" for a while. Instead, we encouraged her to focus on modeling healthy eating behaviors. We also suggested that Gloria and her husband serve Judy appropriate-size portions, rather than letting her help herself. If Judy didn't eat everything on her plate, that was her decision, but she wouldn't get to have seconds of the things she did eat.

When the family returned for their second OWL visit, they reported that the atmosphere at the dinner table had become more peaceful and that Judy seemed ready for the next step. We asked her to take a tiny bite of one new vegetable each week. If she didn't like it, she didn't have to swallow it. Gloria would then reward Judy for her efforts with stickers on a chart. Gradually, Judy would increase the amount and variety of vegetables she ate.

As these efforts progressed, the family created what they called "the vegetable game." Once a week, Gloria would place a new vegetable in Judy's mouth while Judy kept her eyes closed. Judy would chew and swallow the vegetable, then try to answer three questions: Is it cooked or raw? What color is it? What is its name? Afterward, she would draw a picture of the vegetable in her journal.

During her third visit to OWL, Judy reported with pride that she had tried twelve different vegetables and could identify them blindfolded. At this session, we worked on ways to increase physical activity. Over time, Judy discovered that she liked swimming, scootering, soccer, and softball. She considered these activities "fun, not exercise," according to Gloria.

It took some time for Judy to embrace healthy eating and activity habits. "There were some ups and downs, but we stuck with it, knowing she would be so much better off in the long run," Gloria said.

The family's persistence paid off. Judy is now eleven, and her BMI is decreasing at a rate of one to two units each year. "People who haven't seen her in a while talk about how great she looks and how thin she's gotten," Gloria said. "And for the first time, she has a full closet of clothes that she likes." Gloria also sees evidence of her daughter's new sense of self-confidence: "She spends more time looking at herself in the mirror appreciating what she sees." And, much to Gloria's relief, food fights at the dinner table are now a thing of the past.

this, but he just won't listen." Jared begins to bristle. Not wanting the conflict between Jared and his mother to rekindle, I ask Beth what she is most afraid of.

She inhales slowly and says, "I'm afraid that what happened to my father will happen to my son. My dad is obese and diabetic, and he

MICHAEL'S STORY

❖ When fourteen-year-old Michael first came to see us, he suffered from a worrisome combination of weight-related complications. At 5 feet 4 inches tall and 220 pounds, he had very high cholesterol, high triglycerides, insulin resistance, signs of fatty liver, gynecomastia (breast development in a male), shortness of breath when physically active, and poor self-esteem. His lifestyle was very sedentary, and his diet was full of refined starchy foods and concentrated sugars.

Unlike many patients we see in OWL, Michael had largely conflict-free relations with his parents. His big challenge was finding the motivation to change poor eating and physical activity habits. Past weight loss efforts had been halfhearted.

We asked Michael to start by eliminating sugar-sweetened beverages and juices, which contributed about 500 calories to his diet each day. "I didn't want to give up my soda, but that was our first step; that was our baby step," he said. When he came back to see us ten weeks later, he had grown one-half inch and lost ten pounds. With this accomplishment, Michael's motivation increased, and he was willing to make other important changes in his eating habits. He cut down on refined starches such as crackers and bread, ate more fruits and vegetables, and learned to stop eating when he was full. As the weight continued to come off, Michael found it easier to participate in physical activities, and his confidence grew. He enrolled in a karate class and joined a soccer team.

At his most recent clinic visit, Michael was 5 feet 10 inches tall and 155 pounds — representing an astonishing fifteen-unit decrease in BMI. His cholesterol was normal, and the fatty liver had resolved. With a transformed body and renewed self-esteem, Michael, now age nineteen, has gained an appreciation for the value of a healthful lifestyle. "I keep reminding myself of what the last letter of OWL stands for: life. It really is a life thing," he said.

won't take care of himself. I've watched him suffer from all the complications without being able to do anything about it. First a foot and then a leg were amputated. Then he lost his kidneys and needed dialysis. Last year he suffered a stroke, which left him unable to speak clearly."

Jared turns toward her. "Don't worry, Mom. I'll be OK," he assures her.

I feel a growing awareness of what might be causing their conflict. "I understand how concerned you are for your son and how frustrating it can be when he seems not to take your concerns seriously," I say. "You know, I see versions of this basic conflict between parents and their teenage children in our clinic every day."

Addressing Beth, but with Jared listening intently, I explain that most adolescents deny to others, and to themselves, that they have a weight problem. Denial can actually be an appropriate psychological defense against the emotional and sometimes physical pain that many overweight children experience. It helps them deal with feelings of hopelessness, failure, and shame, at least temporarily. Trying to break down a child's resistance by force is often futile, and sometimes psychologically damaging.

The truth is that it can be difficult for anyone, especially children, to lose weight in America today. The world we live in seems to undermine our efforts at every step. Adding insult to injury, images of beauty offered by the media get thinner and thinner, as Americans get heavier and heavier.

Being overweight isn't all Jared's fault. If anyone is to blame, it's a food industry that advertises junk food directly to young kids. It's schools that close budget gaps by peddling fast food and soft drinks to their students. And it's governments that won't build safe parks and recreation centers where children can be physically active.

Beth reflects for a moment, then says, "I know it's not all Jared's fault. And I don't always practice what I preach, especially when it comes to exercise. Perhaps I should ease up on him a bit."

"Perhaps just a bit," I reply. "However, Jared very much needs your help if he is to succeed with weight loss. He has a long way to go before he's fully grown up. With teenagers, in my view, the role of the parent is to support but not to police. We'll discuss this approach in more detail if you and Jared decide to continue in the OWL Program."

Then I say to Jared, "At the beginning of our session, you seemed angry. Can you tell me what you're most angry about?"

His face reddens. "It's just not fair. I hate being fat. I hate how I look."

"You're right, it isn't fair," I say, "although there are a lot of kids and adults, including your mother, who are struggling with their weight, just like you.

"I asked your mother this question, and now I'll ask you. What are you most afraid of?"

"That things will never change," he says. "That no matter what I do, it won't help; I'll always be fat."

"Now that's where I disagree, Jared," I reply.

Thousands of children in OWL and other programs being developed around the country have lost weight and kept it off, sometimes dramatically reversing high blood pressure, high cholesterol, fatty liver, even type 2 diabetes in its early stages.

But first we must welcome them to weight loss. Children need accurate information about their bodies to separate fact from fiction. They need to know that being heavy is not their fault but that there are important reasons to take the situation seriously. And they need to know that there is hope, that they can be successful.

They also need to learn that losing weight can be easy by eating in a way that works with, rather than against, the body's weight control systems (the topic of chapter 3). And they need to discover how good they'll feel giving up TV and getting active (chapter 4). Parents need to understand how psychology affects behavior, and they need age-appropriate techniques to encourage lifestyle change without causing conflict (chapters 5 and 6). Families need a practical, step-by-step approach that they can follow together (chapter 7). Finally, families need to join together to make our communities and our society a healthier place to live (chapter 8).

"In two months," I say to Jared, "you could feel like a new person. In four months, you could look like a new person. And in six months, you could be showing others how you did it.

"So now, it's up to you. Do you want to give the program a try?"

Jared thinks for a moment and nods his head yes.

Beth beams and gives her son a hug and a kiss. "Mom, please, this is so embarrassing," he says. But his smile belies the protest.

PART II

Making Peace
Within Us

3

EATING TO FEEL FULL

I'm hungry."

"But you just ate."

"I'm still hungry. Can I have more? Please?"

It's against a parent's nature to deny his or her child anything that the child really needs, least of all something as fundamentally nurturing as food. After all, food is essential to our survival, and parents' responsibility is to ensure the survival of the next generation. But the food we serve our children is more than a biological necessity. It is an expression of love. So saying no to an extra helping is doubly hard: not only do we feel that we're depriving our children of something that they need to live, but we also feel that we're withholding love.

Imagine meals in which your child eats until she is truly satisfied and still loses weight. Sound like a fantasy? It's not. It is the reality of eating in a way that works with, not against, the body's own weight control systems. It is the way to achieve a healthy weight, peacefully and effectively ending the battle between mind and metabolism within the child and avoiding conflicts between parent and child.

Where do we start? By eating foods that humans evolved to eat over millions of years — foods that digest slowly, providing steady, sustained energy for our metabolism and satisfying our hunger for hours.

Hunger and the energy to run our metabolism are intimately linked. When energy begins to fall, hunger rises so that we'll eat and replenish needed nutrients. When energy is plentiful, hunger falls. What does energy look like inside the body? Picture a tiny fire burning inside each and every cell. These fires release energy, which runs our muscles, sparks our thoughts, and fuels everything that our bodies do. Together, the fires make up our metabolism. The fires have to burn at a steady rate, moment to moment, day to day. Even a brief interruption would be fatal.

So if our metabolism must run constantly, why is it that we don't need to eat all the time, day and night? Why is it unnatural to feel hungry soon after eating? To understand the answers to these questions, it helps to know a bit about how we convert food into energy and into the basic building blocks of our body. Let's roll up our sleeves and take a tour of the inner workings of our digestive system. Afterward, it'll be clear how eating the right foods helps to control hunger, prevent excessive weight gain, and, ultimately, achieve optimal health.

How the Substance of Our Food Becomes the Substance of Our Bodies

The digestion process actually begins before we take the first bite of food. It begins before we even see food, get a whiff of it, or think about it. It begins when the brain senses the need for more energy. Substances in the brain called neuropeptides, along with hormones in the blood, make us feel hungry and prepare the body to receive food. The gastrointestinal tract comes to life with enzymes that break down food. We stop whatever we are doing and look for something to eat.

The gastrointestinal tract may seem like a simple plumbing operation — food in, food out — but digestion has more in common with a

FOOD AS MEDICINE

❖ Humans have a basic biological problem: Our metabolism runs continuously, 24-7. However, the availability of food to fuel our metabolism is unpredictable, and the composition of that food can be highly variable. How are we able to survive during times of scarcity and thrive during times of abundance? The answer is hormones.

Hormones help ration our energy and regulate our weight. Remarkably, most of our hormones respond directly or indirectly to the types and amount of food we eat, transmitting information about the state of our nutrition throughout the body by way of cell receptors. Not enough calories consumed? Over the short term, hormones increase appetite and help convert stored fat into energy. Over the long term, other hormonal changes conserve energy by decreasing metabolic rate. When good nutrition is reestablished, hormones restore metabolic rate to normal, promote optimal growth in children, and maintain reproductive fertility in adults.

It is no coincidence that most drugs that have been used to treat obesity — from thyroid extract in the late nineteenth century to Fen-Phen in the late twentieth century — work through these hormonal pathways. This fact has an astounding implication: if we choose our foods wisely, our diet can potentially do everything that these drugs can do — without the harmful side effects.

computer network than with the kitchen sink. Our stomach and intestines contain about 10 billion nerve cells, the same number as the brain. So in a way, our gastrointestinal tract is as "smart" as our head. This makes sense from an evolutionary perspective: complex thought is a very recent human development, but for hundreds of millions of years, animals have had to extract nourishment from food for survival. In fact, the gastrointestinal tract and the brain are in constant communication. Big bundles of nerve cells (an especially important one is called the vagus nerve) link them together in a vast instant messaging system.

THE BREATH OF FIRE

❖ On a typical day, we eat several pounds of food. The indigestible components of our diet are excreted as stool, and excess water leaves the body as urine. But where does the food we absorb into the body go? Why don't we inevitably gain weight every day? Like a candle burning wax, the body combines the food we eat with the oxygen we inhale, producing energy, water, and carbon dioxide, the end product of our metabolism. Most of the organic matter that we consume leaves the body when we exhale, amounting to many tons in the course a lifetime.

The command center for metabolism and body weight is an ancient part of the brain, no larger than a teaspoon, called the hypothalamus. It constantly surveys the body's nutritional needs, making sure that the proper mixture of nutrients is available to feed our cells and tissues and fuel our metabolism. Working in concert with key hormones such as insulin, the hypothalamus assigns some of the nutrients we eat for immediate use and sets aside the rest to be stored for future needs. The hypothalamus's precise management of our energy supply makes it possible to maintain a relatively stable body weight despite wide swings in the amount and types of food eaten at any one meal.

Almost all of the foods we eat fall into one of three main categories: carbohydrate, which is broken down into the sugar *glucose;* protein, made of *amino acids;* and fat, composed of various *fatty acids.* Just like a candle burning wax, our bodies can transform these nutrients into usable energy, called *calories.* Our bodies also use some of the foods we eat for the growth and repair of tissue. Amino acids extracted from the protein in foods are recombined to form other kinds of protein, the main building blocks for muscles, organs, connective tissue, and other important structures. Fatty acids are used to form the membrane that surrounds each cell in the body. Every molecule that moves in or out of a cell — all communication between cells — takes place through this vital membrane. For this reason, the types of fats we eat can have a profound effect on our nervous system, immune function, and general health. What happens to the food we eat that isn't needed to fuel our metabolism or build tissue? Unfortunately, the body has no way to dispose of these extra calories. Instead, they're converted into fat and stored.

Fiber, the indigestible component of plants, is best known for keeping our bowels regular, but it has many other important functions. For one, it stays in our stomachs for a while, thereby helping us to stay full. Fiber also carries with it many different vitamins, minerals, and phytochemicals. Vitamins are essential for the hundreds of biochemical reactions that take place in the body, moment to moment. Minerals maintain salt balance inside and outside the cells. Phytochemicals (literally, plant chemicals) are substances that give plants color, taste, and a variety of beneficial health properties. Some phytochemicals and vitamins are antioxidants, compounds that help prevent sparks from our metabolic fire from doing harm.

Let's see what happens when we have a snack, say, of almonds and dates. We taste the richness of the almonds and the sweetness of the dates. We savor the almonds' crunchiness and the dates' chewiness. This sensory information travels up to the brain and down to the rest of the digestive tract through nerves, signaling that food is on the way.

Chewing breaks food down into smaller pieces. Enzymes in saliva begin to digest the carbohydrates, breaking them down into glucose. After a few seconds, we swallow, and the esophagus escorts our snack into the stomach with a wave of muscular contractions.

The stomach then churns the food, furthering its mechanical digestion. Nerves in the stomach can actually sense what kinds of nutrients are present in the food, adding this information to the instant messaging system that connects the gastrointestinal tract and the brain. Enzymes in the stomach are released, beginning the digestion of protein into amino acids.

When the stomach has finished its job, the food is released into the small intestine, where most of the digestion takes place. The body carefully controls the amount of food it lets into the small intestine: admitting too much at a time would overwhelm the body's ability to digest the food; admitting too little would keep us from getting enough nourishment.

At this point, a whole new set of powerful enzymes enters the small intestine, including those that break down fats. Cells that line the small intestine absorb glucose, amino acids, and fatty acids and release them into the bloodstream. As blood sugar rises, the pancreas responds by secreting more insulin. This hormone is best known for ferrying glucose out of the blood and into energy-hungry cells. But it also tells the entire body that nutrients are coming in — prepare to feast.

From Caveman to Carl's Jr.

Clearly, not every meal that we eat is a perfect balance of nutrients. But that's all right. The body does a remarkable job of adapting to a variety of different diets and still satisfying its need for a continuous supply of fuel. Human metabolism adjusts to periods of feasting and fasting. If we gorge at one meal, the body will compensate by suppressing our appetite at the next meal. If we fast, our appetite will increase, ensuring that we eat more than usual when the fast ends.

Our metabolism has evolved over millions of years to allow us to get by on many kinds of foods. Traditional peoples who live in the Arctic eat lots of fats from fish and virtually no carbohydrates for much of the year. Traditional peoples living in the tropics eat a lot of fruits, vegetables, and other carbohydrates. We do beautifully well on a great variety of foods, with a wide range of nutrients, as long as we're eating a natural diet.

What kinds of foods were humans designed to eat? Let's imagine we are living in the Stone Age. We eat foods we can gather, such as leafy vegetables, root vegetables, beans, fruits, and nuts, or foods we can catch (when we're lucky), such as fish. These are whole foods. They take time to eat. They digest slowly and sustain our metabolism.

Today, however, the largest source of calories for most children (and many adults) is food that doesn't exist in nature at all: highly re-fined carbohydrates, such as white bread, prepared breakfast cereals, white rice, potato chips, cookies, candy, and, of course, sugary drinks. These foods, which have a high glycemic index, are extremely easy to overeat. They raise blood sugar too rapidly, setting in motion a chain of events that make it hard to avoid gaining too much weight. Let's take a look at what the glycemic index is and why it is important to your weight and your health.

High–Glycemic Index Foods, Overeating, and Obesity

All carbohydrates are composed of sugar, either in single units or short chains called *simple sugars,* or in long chains, called *starches.* Tradi-tionally, simple sugars were considered unhealthy. Located at the top of the government's original Food Guide Pyramid, they were meant to be eaten sparingly. Starchy foods, such as bread, rice, and potatoes, were considered healthy. Placed at the base of the pyramid, they were to be eaten in abundance (see Figure 3.1).

Unfortunately, this notion is completely wrong. When a starchy food is refined (by stripping the fiber off of whole grains and milling them into fine flour), the body can digest it into sugar quite literally in seconds. Try this: Take a bite of a bagel, chew it well, and hold it in your mouth for a few moments. You'll notice that it begins to taste sweet. Bagels aren't usually made with added sugar; the sweet taste comes from sugar molecules breaking off from the starch under the digestive action of saliva. Once a refined starchy food is swallowed and moves down the digestive tract, it melts into sugar. A bagel and a bowl of sugar may taste different in the mouth, but below the neck, they are virtually the same.

Back in the 1970s, David Jenkins, a gastroenterologist at the Uni-versity of Toronto, decided to test the effects of carbohydrate-contain-ing foods on blood sugar and insulin. He and his colleagues had volun-teers eat about two ounces of carbohydrates from various foods and

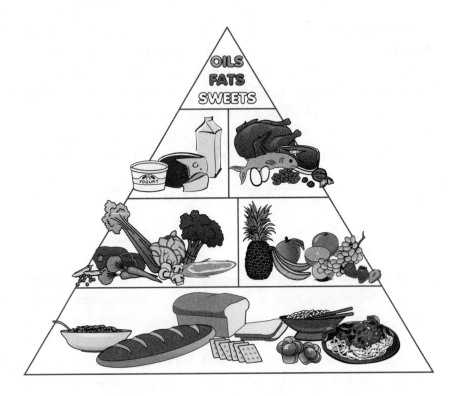

Figure 3.1 The Original Food Guide Pyramid

then measured changes in blood sugar concentration over the next two hours. On a separate day, each of the subjects consumed the same amount of carbohydrates from glucose. The researchers then assigned each of these foods a number based on how much it raised blood sugar compared to glucose: the faster the rate of digestion and absorption, the higher the number.

Jenkins unveiled this numerical value system to the world in 1981 as the *glycemic index.* It was a revelation. Some of the foods commonly thought to be healthy, such as potatoes, raced through the digestive tract even faster than table sugar. White rice, corn, and packaged breakfast cereals (even unsweetened cereals) also had a very high glycemic index. In contrast, some of the foods made up primarily of sugars (such as whole fruit) had a low glycemic index, because it takes time for the digestive tract to break down most intact, unprocessed foods. The glycemic index rendered the distinction between simple and complex carbohydrates meaningless.

In 1997, Walter Willett and colleagues at Harvard adapted the glycemic index to apply more directly to real-life serving sizes. After all, we don't always eat the same amount of carbohydrates from one food to the next. Whereas a potato has a lot of carbohydrates, a serving of carrots has very little. So the *glycemic load* tells us how blood sugar will change after eating typical portions of foods.

The glycemic effect of foods has been used for years to help people with diabetes keep their blood sugar and insulin levels under control. But I became intrigued by its potential for helping overweight children manage their weight. The prevailing recommendation that these children reduce the amount of fat in their diets wasn't working well, but doctors were wary of putting children on more restrictive diets. Extreme diets, by their very nature, involve deprivation — of calories and often of nutrients. This can be risky for anybody, but for a growing, developing child, it can do harm physically and psychologically.

When we looked at the glycemic values of foods, we noticed an interesting pattern. The foods with the lowest glycemic values were more natural and nutritious than those with the highest values. They were fruits, vegetables, beans, nuts, and whole grains. The foods with the highest glycemic values were mainly refined and highly processed carbohydrates: chips, cakes, cookies, sugary breakfast cereals, and sodas. These were the foods that had become a growing part of the American diet since the 1960s — the very period when childhood obesity increased to epidemic proportions.

We decided to test the effects of high-glycemic and low-glycemic meals on hormones and hunger in 12 obese teenage boys. On separate days, we gave these boys three different breakfasts with identical calories but different glycemic values. The high-glycemic breakfast was instant oatmeal with a little milk and sugar. The medium-glycemic breakfast was oatmeal made from steel-cut oats — the kind that Grandma used to make. Oatmeal made from steel-cut oats takes longer to cook and to digest than instant oatmeal. The low-glycemic

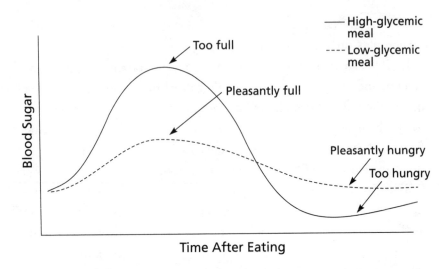

Figure 3.2 Changes in Blood Sugar After Low-
and High-Glycemic Meals

breakfast was a vegetable omelet with fruit that had a bit more protein and fat than the oatmeals. Afterward, the boys could eat whatever they wanted from a large snack platter. Meanwhile, we tested the boys' blood for glucose, insulin, and other hormones.

As expected, blood sugar and insulin rose a lot after the instant oatmeal, a moderate amount after the steel-cut oats, and only a little after the omelet. But what goes up must come down: blood sugar fell to very low levels, even below where it had started, several hours after the high-glycemic instant oatmeal but not after the other breakfasts (see Figure 3.2). This blood sugar "crash" was severe enough to cause a surge in adrenaline, also called epinephrine, a powerful hormone released during times of stress. And how does someone with low blood sugar and surging adrenaline feel? Tired, irritable, and hungry.

When we measured how much the boys subsequently ate, the results were startling. They consumed 600 to 700 calories more after the high-glycemic instant oatmeal than after the other two breakfasts. If only part of these excess calories were eaten meal after meal, day after day, it could explain much of the increased rate of obesity in the United States over the past forty years, as the amount of high-glycemic foods in our diets has increased.

What kinds of foods do we crave when our blood sugar is low? Refined starchy foods and concentrated sugars — high-glycemic foods that raise blood sugar quickly but set up the next ride on the blood sugar roller coaster. To make matters worse, the high insulin levels resulting from a high-glycemic meal temporarily shut off the release of fatty acids from fat tissue, making it even harder to burn off those excess calories.

HOW SWEET IS IT?

❖ In a classic experiment from the 1970s, scientists gave subjects two drinks — one sweetened with sugar, the other sweetened artificially. Initially, the subjects couldn't taste any difference between them and liked both equally. Then the scientists gave them a substance that mimics the effect of low blood sugar, and a very interesting thing happened: they developed a strong preference for the sugar-sweetened drink and perceived it as sweeter. The brain could somehow distinguish between sugar, which raises blood sugar rapidly, and artificial sweetener, which doesn't raise blood sugar at all. This experiment shows how our biology (for example, low blood sugar) can affect our psychology (the desire for something with a high glycemic index) and, conversely, how our behavior (eating something with a high glycemic index) can affect our biology (blood sugar).

More than a dozen similar studies have confirmed our findings that people are less hungry, feel fuller, and eat less following low-glycemic meals than high-glycemic meals. But what happens over the long term? It's no secret that most people who go on low-calorie diets eventually gain back the weight they lose and then some. One explanation for such poor results is that each of us has a body weight set point (as mentioned in chapter 1) that is defended by fundamental biological mechanisms. According to this theory, when we cut back on calories, the body rebels by slowing down metabolism and increasing hunger. So it becomes progressively harder to burn off calories and resist overeating.

To find out if low-glycemic meals could quiet this rebellion, we studied overweight and obese young adults on low-calorie diets that had either a high-glycemic or a low-glycemic load. The two diets were designed to produce a 10 percent weight loss (about twenty pounds) in ten weeks. After weight loss, subjects in both groups showed a slowdown in metabolism, but metabolic rate decreased significantly more among those eating the high-glycemic diet — a difference of 80 calories per day. Over a year, these 80 calories per day could amount to an extra eight-pound weight gain. In addition, subjects on the high-glycemic diet reported greater hunger. The bottom line? Low-glycemic eating may alter the body weight set point, making it easier to lose weight and keep it off.

Another intriguing finding from this study was that risk factors for diabetes and heart disease improved more on the low-glycemic diet, even though this diet had more fat, more cholesterol, and more salt than the high-glycemic diet. Blood pressure and triglycerides (the amount of fat in the blood) decreased more on the low-glycemic diet. C-reactive protein, a newly identified risk factor that indicates chronic inflammation, dropped by 50 percent on the low-glycemic diet but remained essentially unchanged on the high-glycemic diet. In addition, insulin resistance, a condition in which the body fails to respond properly to insulin, decreased more than twice as much on the low-glycemic diet compared to the high-glycemic diet. Insulin resistance is one of the most important risk factors for type 2 diabetes, the kind of diabetes that occurs with obesity.

We have extended these findings in studies lasting up to one year with overweight or obese children, teenagers, and adults. For these studies, we gave one group a low-glycemic diet that was higher in fat and another group a low-fat diet that was higher in glycemic load. We instructed the low-fat group to cut back on food by about 500 calories per day, in accordance with conventional recommendations. In contrast, we allowed the low-glycemic group to eat until they were satisfied and to snack when hungry. Of course, there is no violating the basic laws of physics: to lose weight, one must take in fewer calories or burn off more calories. However, we theorized that individuals eating a low-glycemic diet would feel less hungry and decrease their food intake naturally, without being told to restrict calories. If this method worked, it would be especially great for children, helping to avoid power struggles between parents and kids over when and how much to eat. Indeed, one long-standing concern with calorie-restricted diets in adolescents is the possibility of precipitating an eating disorder, in effect substituting one serious disease for another.

In the children's study, those on the low-glycemic diet (without calorie restriction) lost about seven pounds more than those on the low-fat diet after an average of four months. In the adolescent study, those on the low-glycemic diet lost ten pounds of body fat more than those on the low-fat diet after one year. In the adult study, those on the low-glycemic diet had significantly better triglycerides and plasminogen activator inhibitor-1, a newly identified heart disease risk factor that increases the likelihood of forming blood clots in the arteries.

Based on these and other clinical trials, it appeared that the glycemic index of foods had an important effect on body weight, as well as on the risks for important medical complications. But a nagging question remained: was it the glycemic index that made the difference, or was it some other attribute of the foods that could vary along with their glycemic index, such as fiber content, taste, or energy density (calories per bite)?

We set out to answer this question by studying laboratory rodents, feeding them diets that were much more strictly controlled than would be possible in studies with humans. We fed one group of rats a diet with a high glycemic index and another group a diet with a low

DILLON'S STORY

❖ Not all the patients I see in OWL do well right from the start. Unhealthful lifestyle habits, even for children, don't always shift overnight. And sometimes psychological issues or family dynamics require attention before progress can be made. But for motivated families with a simple lack of nutritional knowledge, just a few sessions can be all that it takes. This was the case for Dillon and his family.

We first saw Dillon when he was four years old. Dillon had always been big, but his weight had recently become a hindrance to him in karate and other physical activities. His mother described Dillon as having an enormous appetite, "with no shutoff valve." The family tried to keep Dillon constantly distracted because when he was not busy, he'd want to eat. His mother, who'd struggled with her own weight all her life, had put Dillon on what she believed to be a healthy low-fat diet. Despite her efforts, Dillon's weight had climbed to 63 pounds; at 3 feet 7 inches tall, he had a BMI of 24, way off the charts for such a young child.

Dillon was eating what had conventionally been considered a "healthy low-fat diet." It was also a very high-glycemic diet. He had a banana and low-fat waffles for breakfast; crackers for a morning snack; a peanut butter and jelly sandwich (light on the peanut butter) for lunch; crackers and fruit for an afternoon snack; lean meat, rice or potatoes, and a vegetable for dinner; and a fat-free Popsicle for dessert.

To Dillon's mother's dismay, we suggested that she abandon the low-fat diet, cook the family's vegetables in a generous amount of olive oil, and put more peanut butter on Dillon's sandwich. We also suggested that she emphasize lower-glycemic fruits (apple instead of banana, for example) and add some protein to his breakfast. Finally, we advised her to cut back on refined grains, including waffles, crackers, white rice, and potatoes. After some initial reluctance, she agreed to give the low-glycemic eating plan a try.

When the family returned just two months later, the results were dramatic. Dillon had lost six pounds — 10 percent of his body weight — and grown half an inch. Generally speaking, young children needn't actually lose any weight to deal successfully with a weight problem. By holding weight constant for a period of time, or even slowing down the rate of weight gain, most can grow out of the problem. Indeed, a rapid weight loss may indicate an excessively restrictive diet that can be unhealthy for anyone, especially young children. However, Dillon's mother reported that he was eating three solid meals and several snacks a day and had markedly decreased hunger and noticeably improved energy, all reassuring signs.

Two months later, Dillon was still losing weight. His mother had to buy him new pants because the old ones were too loose. In addition, she reported that Dillon had better balance and coordination during karate and improved self-confidence.

After ten months, Dillon had grown two inches and lost a total of ten pounds, showing continuing improvement in energy level, physical abilities, and confidence. And now, almost two years after starting OWL, Dillon's BMI is approaching the normal range for a six-year-old. His mother had to buy him yet another set of new clothes, but she didn't mind at all.

glycemic index, carefully maintaining the same total body weight in the two groups. After about four months (about ten years to a human), the high-glycemic group had almost twice as much fat as the low-glycemic group, even though both groups had the same total weight. Moreover, almost all of the extra fat was in the belly area, where fat poses the greatest risk for health complications. The high-glycemic group also had three times more fat in the blood and severe abnormalities in the cells that make insulin. So glycemic index really does influence body fat and other health risk factors by itself, independent of other aspects of the diet.

Now imagine if we had a drug that could convert belly fat to muscle and reduce the risk for complications of obesity. The news would make the front page of the *New York Times,* the stock price for the company holding the drug patent would soar, millions of prescriptions

A LETTER FROM MARIA'S MOM

❖ Like Dillon, Maria had been eating a low-fat, very high-glycemic diet. When she first came to see us at age six, she was 3 feet 9 inches tall and weighed 72 pounds, placing her well above the 95th percentile for BMI. We suggested some simple dietary changes: avoiding snacks containing just refined carbohydrates (chips, crackers, pretzels, Popsicles) and increasing vegetables, whole fruits, nut butters, and healthy protein. After five months in OWL, her mother wrote me this letter:

Dear Dr. Ludwig,

I was very hesitant to come to the OWL clinic. I was thinking I was this terrible mother and my daughter's self-esteem and confidence would drop dramatically if I were to bring her there. Well, since coming to see you, it has done just the opposite. She is not shy as she used to be. She's more outgoing and talkative, but most of all, she's happy, and she feels good about herself. The last time we were there, she had lost about eleven pounds and grown half an inch. She will be starting first grade in ten days, and today we bought jeans for school. These are the first pair of pants I could buy her that had a normal button and zipper instead of an elastic band. Everyone around us cannot believe the change physically and emotionally in her. I do not think kids will be calling her names like last year. We will continue to eat healthy and stay active!

would be written — and then in about five years, if the past is any guide, the drug would be taken off the market due to unexpected life-threatening complications. Now imagine that we had a diet that could do these things safely. Although some controversy still exists (see page 70) and more research is needed, the latest research suggests that we do have such a diet and that it actually tastes good.

High-Glycemic Foods and Your Family's Health

The link between high-glycemic foods and disease has been examined in dozens of epidemiological studies in which large numbers of individuals have been followed over the long term while consuming their normal diets. My colleagues at Harvard who conduct the Nurses' Health Study found that women eating a high-glycemic diet have substantially greater risks for type 2 diabetes, heart disease, and stroke regardless of body weight. This means that a low-glycemic diet could improve health in two ways: by promoting weight loss and by protecting against serious illnesses at any body weight.

High-glycemic foods may also be linked to another major life-threatening disease: cancer. People eating a high-glycemic diet produce more insulin than those eating a low-glycemic diet. Insulin is a key hormone regulating blood sugar, but it is also a potent growth factor that could, at high concentrations, stimulate cells to proliferate excessively and, at least in theory, undergo transformation into cancer. In studies from the United States, Canada, Italy, and Switzerland, a high-glycemic diet has been linked to breast, endometrial, ovarian, prostate, stomach, pancreatic, and colorectal cancer in adults, although the topic remains controversial among scientists, and much more research is needed.

A high-glycemic diet may carry other risks, especially for children. As we saw earlier, a high-glycemic breakfast can result in low blood sugar and surging adrenaline levels a few hours later. Remember, adrenaline is an emergency stress hormone whose job is to prepare the body for a potentially life-threatening stress. So how might your ten-year-old son feel sitting in a social studies class at school several hours after eating a bagel and fat-free cream cheese for breakfast? Would he be sitting quietly, concentrating and behaving well? Or might he appear distracted and fidgety? If he had an underlying tendency, perhaps he might act as if he had attention deficit hyperactivity disorder (ADHD). Clearly, ADHD is a complex disorder with many genetic and environmental causes. However, parents in the OWL Program sometimes report that their children's behavior improves dramatically once they start eating low-glycemic foods, even before they've lost any weight. Is it really so surprising that the foods we eat could affect our minds as well as our bodies?

Nancy, the mother of a six-year-old girl, said on her second visit to OWL, "You've given me my child back!" In the past, her daughter had frequent temper tantrums late in the afternoon as Nancy was trying to prepare dinner. Any little thing seemed to set her off, and once she got started, the only way to settle her down was with food. At those times, Nancy had to put family dinner preparation on hold and make something quick for her daughter to eat, such as macaroni and cheese. Now, with a low-glycemic snack after school, her mood remains stable all afternoon, she plays quietly while Nancy cooks, and everyone dines together.

FOOD FOR THOUGHT

❖ Several recently published studies highlight the impact of food on mental function. David Benton at the University of Wales in the United Kingdom gave undergraduates cereal-based breakfasts that were either low or high glycemic index and then examined their ability to recall words. Students who ate the low-glycemic breakfast had better cognitive performance throughout the morning and were able to remember 50 percent more abstract words after three and a half hours. In a study from Toronto, patients with diabetes were given low- or high-glycemic breakfasts. Over the next two hours, those having the low-glycemic meal showed significantly better working memory (ability to hold words in the mind for current use), selective attention (ability to filter out distractions), and executive function (ability to plan, think abstractly, and initiate appropriate action). Eating well helps us think clearly, and clear thinking may help us choose our foods wisely.

The Fast Track to Weight Gain

Many high-glycemic carbohydrates became staples of the American diet over the past four decades because we thought they were healthy. Bread, rice, and potatoes enjoyed star billing at the base of the Food Guide Pyramid as foods that should make up the bulk of our diet. Fats, along with sugars, appeared at the top of the pyramid as foods we should eat sparingly. Some studies linked dietary fats with various health problems, including heart disease and cancer (although these studies often didn't distinguish adequately between good fats and bad). So we cut fats out of our diet and replaced them with carbohydrates. Food manufacturers eagerly met the increased demand for carbohydrates with cheap, high-glycemic products such as chips, crackers, cookies, and other refined starches and sweets labeled "reduced fat" or "fat-free." We guiltlessly ate them and served them to our children because they tasted good and seemed wholesome. But most were the nutritional equivalent of table sugar.

Our love affair with high-glycemic carbs was also a matter of convenience. Most packaged foods that can be microwaved or otherwise rendered ready to eat in minutes have a high glycemic value. So does fast food. Many people think of fast food as being loaded with fats, but it actually contains an even greater amount of high-glycemic carbohydrates: the hamburger bun, fries, soda, cookies, and even ketchup are all loaded with refined starches and concentrated sugars.

Few outside the industry would argue that fast food is good for you, but until recently there were no studies that looked at whether eating fast food on a regular basis affects body weight or any health outcome. For this reason, we examined 3,000 young adults over a fifteen-year period. The results were more disturbing than we had expected. Individuals consuming fast food more than twice a week gained an extra ten pounds, and insulin resistance increased twice as fast, compared to those eating fast food less than once a week. Moreover, this study began in the 1980s, when fast food consumption was much lower than it is now. What about children today, eating fast food four times a week or more? Did somebody say Happy Meals? These are very sad meals indeed.

SLOW FOOD

❖ Fast food has just about the worst imaginable combination of dietary factors, including massive portion size, high energy density, huge glycemic load, large amounts of partially hydrogenated (trans) and saturated fats, minimal amounts of fiber, and few vitamins and minerals — each independently related to risk for obesity, diabetes, or heart disease. And if that isn't enough, fast food also seems to promote weight gain by its very nature: it's designed to be eaten fast. A child can easily consume almost an entire day's calorie requirements from a fast food meal in just a few minutes, before the body has a chance to recognize and respond to the incoming calories.

❖ As we saw earlier in this chapter, the gastrointestinal tract communicates with the brain through nerves and hormones about the nature of the foods we consume. But it can take time, twenty to thirty minutes, for these "satiety signals" to be sent and for us to know when we've had enough. For this reason, eating slowly is an important way to avoid overeating. So whether you're having a burger and fries or a fine French meal, slow down. You'll get more enjoyment during the meal, you probably won't feel overstuffed after the meal, and you may notice a smaller waistline before long.

Low-Glycemic Eating: The Perfect Compromise Between Low Fat and Low Carb

For much of the past thirty-five years, most people trying to lose weight have followed a low-fat diet. This seemed to make sense: if you

IT GETS YOU IN THE GUT

❖ One of the most common, though least recognized, complications of obesity is fatty liver. As many as 1 in 3 overweight children and 1 in 2 obese adults have evidence of excessive fat accumulation in the liver. In some individuals, for unclear reasons, this condition can cause progressive liver damage, resulting in cirrhosis and liver failure. Recent research suggests that glycemic index can play a role in this process. Among apparently healthy Italians, individuals consuming diets highest in glycemic index were twice as likely to have fatty liver compared to those consuming diets lower in glycemic index.

don't want fat *on* your body, don't put fat *in* your body. There was one problem, however: it didn't work. The proportion of fat in our diet has decreased dramatically since the 1960s, but the obesity epidemic has exploded. In fact, research from our laboratory and from others has shown that the relative amount of fat in the diet has little or no effect on body weight.

Several years ago, the pendulum swung very far in the other direction with the enormous popularity of low-carb diets. These diets do produce more weight loss than low-fat diets, but only temporarily. After one year, people following both types of diets gain back nearly all of the weight they lose. These approaches ultimately fail because our bodies and our minds rebel against severe restriction of any major nutrient, whether fat or carbohydrate. (How long do you want to keep eating that bacon double cheeseburger, hold the bun, thank you?) When deprived, our bodies hold on to calories with increasing tenacity, and willpower dissolves.

Most low-calorie diets are symptomatic treatment at best. They work for a while, but they don't get at the underlying causes of over-

SEEING IS BELIEVING

❖ The eye is one of the most sensitive parts of the body to high blood sugar. That's why loss of vision is one of the most common, and feared, complications of poorly controlled diabetes. Might the excessive swings in blood sugar resulting from a high-glycemic diet affect vision, even in individuals without diabetes? According to a recent study, the answer is yes. Among women in the Nurses' Health Study, the likelihood of developing macular degeneration (the most common cause of blindness over age fifty) was almost three times greater in those consuming high- compared to low-glycemic diets.

eating. It's like treating an asthma attack with an inhaler. Breathing may get better temporarily, but if the underlying precipitants aren't addressed (that dusty bedroom rug or the relative at home who smokes), the asthma attacks will continue. Inhaler overuse may actually exacerbate the problem.

To have the best chance of achieving real, long-term weight loss, we need an abundance of truly nourishing foods. Unlike low-calorie diets, low-glycemic eating does not produce deprivation, for the body or the mind. It works with, rather than against, the underlying biology that governs body weight, while incorporating the widest possible range of foods. We needn't deprive ourselves of nutrients or restrict entire classes of foods, although some diet books advise this approach. Why waste the effort on dietary measures that don't provide long-term results? Deprivation isn't necessary to lose weight, and it's definitely not desirable for children.

The Right Carbs, the Right Protein, the Right Fats

Earlier in this chapter, we saw how foods can affect our hormones and hunger in very different ways. From this perspective, restricting ourselves to low-calorie foods or skipping meals doesn't make sense if we wind up feeling excessively hungry. In the battle between mind and metabolism, metabolism usually wins.

So let's do away with calorie counting, food scales, and eating by the numbers. Let's give up diets that restrict the *quantity* of the foods we can eat or that eliminate entire nutrient groups. The key to low-glycemic eating (see Figure 3.3) is to focus on the *quality* of the carbohydrates, protein, and fats and let our bodies do the rest. By eating the right foods, in the right combinations, we will stay full longer, and fewer calories will go farther. (Refer to the shopping list beginning on page 307 as a guide to foods with healthy carbohydrates, protein, and fats.)

Carbohydrate: Almost all of the carbohydrates in our diets come from plants: whole grains, fruits, berries, leafy vegetables, root vegetables, peas, beans, and nuts. These foods nourish us with the richness of nature. In their natural states, carbohydrates almost always have a low or moderate glycemic index, releasing their sugars into our bodies in a slow and sustained way. In addition, they usually have a low energy density. Research by Barbara Rolls at Penn State University shows that meals with a low energy density help people feel full with fewer calories. Eat an abundant amount of carbohydrates with a low or moderate glycemic index. Problems occur when carbohydrates are excessively processed: whole grains pulverized into flour and the fiber stripped away, whole apples turned into juice, sugar cane or sugar beets used to make table sugar. White bread, white rice, highly processed breakfast cereals, crackers, cookies, chips, and concentrated sugars typically have a high glycemic index. There is no need to get rid of them entirely, just limit them to a side dish or small dessert as part of an otherwise balanced meal.

BROKEN GRAIN, WEIGHT GAIN, CHEST PAIN

❖ Can eating too much white bread, processed breakfast cereal, or other highly refined carbohydrate fatten your child and give you a heart attack? Sound preposterous? Actually, the link is quite clear. Intact, "unbroken" grains contain myriad substances known to prevent disease and promote optimal health. In study after study, fiber from whole grains has among the strongest protective effects of all dietary factors. Finely milled whole grain flours still have the fiber and other beneficial substances of unbroken grains, although some of the vitamins and antioxidants are more susceptible to degradation. And since the structure has been disrupted, the glycemic index is markedly increased, approaching that of table sugar. In making white flour, virtually all of the beneficial nutrients are removed, leaving just the "naked starch." In fact, refined grain products have so little nutritional value that the government mandates that most such products be fortified by adding back a few of the missing vitamins. However, fortification is an extremely poor substitute for the original: consumption of refined grains is associated with increased risks for heart disease and diabetes.

Protein: Amino acids from protein are necessary for growth, tissue repair, and the proper functioning of all chemical reactions in the body. But protein plays a special role in body weight management. Protein slows down digestion in the gastrointestinal tract. As a result, carbohydrates eaten with protein at the same meal are digested more slowly than carbohydrates eaten alone. In addition, protein stimulates the release of glucagon, a hormone that helps the body release stored fuels such as fat when blood sugar begins to fall, balancing the effect of insulin. In part for these reasons, high-protein foods are often particularly "satiating" (filling).

Many people wonder whether children can get enough protein without eating meat. In fact, vegetarians (who eat dairy and eggs) or

ANIMAL OR VEGETABLE?

❖ Humans are omnivorous and have evolved eating meat as a component of our diets. However, industrial farm animals are very different from the wild animals our ancestors hunted or fished. They have much more saturated fats and are often treated with antibiotics and growth-promoting substances. Industrial dairy cows are milked intensively during pregnancy, leading to high concentrations of hormones in milk and other dairy products. Some of these hormones may trigger early puberty, acne, reproductive disorders, and perhaps even cancer.

Some people have ethical concerns about the poor conditions in which industrial animals are raised or about eating animals at all. Others are concerned about the environment. The fact is, it's not good for our health, or for the planet, for us to eat meat at every meal, as discussed by Michael Jacobson in his book *Six Arguments for a Greener Diet*. For this reason, we offer vegetarian options for all of the recipes in chapter 9.

vegans (who eat no animal products at all) can get perfectly adequate amounts of protein with proper planning. Soybean products such as tofu are excellent sources of protein, although these foods can be a stretch for some kids at first. Among animal products, red meat usually has much more saturated fat (the type of fat that raises cholesterol) than fish or chicken.

Fat: Since fats have twice the calories per ounce as carbohydrates or protein, most calorie-restricted diets have advocated reducing this major nutrient as much as possible. However, fats can be filling; like protein, they slow down digestion, reducing the surge in blood sugar that occurs after eating high-glycemic carbohydrates. And since fats are tasty, they can make vegetables a whole lot more appealing to children. So throw away the fat-free dressing and low-fat cooking spray.

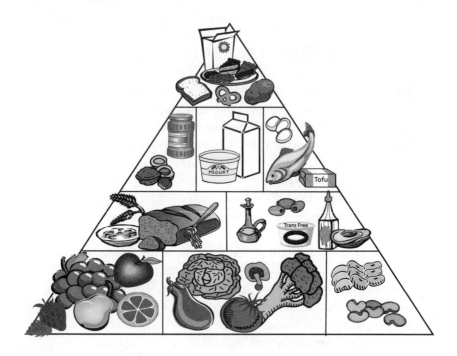

Figure 3.3 A Low-Glycemic Food Pyramid

Go ahead and give your child a liberal serving of nut butter on toast (whole grain, of course) for breakfast, an avocado dip with chips (or better yet, raw vegetables) for an afternoon snack, and broccoli sautéed in olive oil for dinner.

Like carbohydrates, all fats are not created equal. The best are unsaturated oils, which are liquid at room temperature. Saturated fats, chiefly from animal products, tend to raise cholesterol and can increase the risk for heart disease when consumed in excessive amounts. Partially hydrogenated fats (also called trans fats) are the closest things to poison in our food supply. Almost all food additives, such as preservatives, artificial colors, and artificial sweeteners, are added to food products in trace amounts. In contrast, partially hydrogenated fats are found in fast food and a long list of processed, packaged foods in huge quantities. Virtually nonexistent in nature, these unnatural compounds penetrate our tissues, disrupt cell membrane function, and al-

---

BEAUTY IS MORE THAN SKIN-DEEP

❖ The glycemic values of foods may make the difference between the occasional pimple and a face covered with acne. According to one Australian study, teenagers who switched to a low-glycemic diet had fewer pimples than teenagers who continued eating their normal diet.

---

ter hormonal responses. Whereas unsaturated fats actually decrease the risks for diabetes and heart disease, partially hydrogenated fats increase the risks for these and other chronic health conditions and, according to preliminary data, may promote weight gain.

I KNOW WHAT you're thinking: How am I going to get my child to eat all these unfamiliar foods? And even if I could, how am I going to find the time to prepare them? Don't worry. In part III, we will show you, step by step, how to change your family's eating habits gradually, making the transition to healthier meals just as hundreds of families in the OWL Program have done.

The Eight Principles of Low-Glycemic Eating

1. Eat an abundance of nonstarchy vegetables, beans, and fruits. (Temperate fruits such as apples, pears, peaches, and berries tend to have a lower glycemic index than tropical fruits such as banana and mangoes.)
2. Eat grains in the least processed state possible: "unbroken," such as whole kernel bread, brown rice, and whole barley, millet, and wheat berries; or traditionally processed, such as stone-ground bread, steel-cut oats, and natural granola or muesli breakfast cereals.

3. Limit refined grain products and potatoes to small side dishes.

4. Limit concentrated sweets to occasional treats, reduce fruit juice to no more than one cup a day, and completely eliminate sugar-sweetened drinks.

5. Eat a healthful type of protein at most meals.

6. Choose healthful fats, such as olive oil, nuts (almonds, walnuts, pecans), and avocados. Limit saturated fats from dairy and other animal products. Completely eliminate partially hydrogenated fats (trans fats), present in fast food and many packaged foods.

7. Have three meals and one or two snacks each day, and don't skip breakfast.

8. Eat slowly and stop when full.

CONTROVERSIES

❖ The glycemic index has been the subject of much controversy in the past decade. Many official organizations around the world recommend a low-glycemic diet for health promotion and disease prevention, but no major professional association in the United States has fully embraced the concept. Two main criticisms have been raised about the glycemic index, and both are true — in part. Let's have a look at the arguments.

1. Some high calorie foods, such as ice cream, have a low glycemic index. (True)

So people on a low-glycemic diet should eat lots of it? (Unfortunately not)

No single nutritional concept could ever fully define a healthful diet. Not even the most ardent advocates of a low-fat diet would recommend drinking Coke all day because it's fat-free. When considering groups of similar foods (bread products, for example), the lower–glycemic index items tend to be the healthiest. However, we need to use a bit of common sense as well.

2. Individual foods can affect blood sugar differently when eaten alone or as part of a complete meal. (True)

So there's really no point in considering glycemic index. (False)

The amount that blood sugar rises after eating a carbohydrate-containing food can be reduced by combining the food with protein or fats. That's why we recommend having half a bagel with peanut butter rather than a whole bagel by itself. However, high–glycemic index foods consistently produce higher blood sugar levels than low–glycemic index foods, whether the foods are eaten alone or in a complete meal. And many studies — involving thousands of individuals preparing and combining foods in their usual ways — have shown that glycemic index has a major impact on risks for diabetes, heart disease, and other obesity-related conditions.

The bottom line is this: many factors combine to make a healthful diet, including calories, energy density, content of vitamins and minerals, and quality of fats and protein. When considering glycemic index, let's not "eat by the numbers" — it's not necessary, and it takes the fun out of eating. Instead, as Marion Nestle says in her book *What to Eat,* "The glycemic index alerts you to the good things that happen when you eat foods . . . [like] fruits, vegetables and whole grains . . . The glycemic index also alerts you to the undesirable effects of eating lots of starchy processed foods . . . and foods high in added sugars."

A Bonus for Kids

Many parents I see are understandably concerned about putting their children on a diet. Pediatricians share this concern. They worry about the risks of depriving children of foods that they need for growth and development. They worry about causing conflict within the family, as well-meaning parents say no to extra helpings. They worry about the psychological repercussions: Some children might feel blamed for their appearance, singled out, and punished, causing shame and eroding self-esteem. Others might become obsessed with losing weight, increasing the risk of developing an eating disorder.

IT'S NEVER TOO SOON TO START

❖ According to conventional thinking, genes establish an individual's lifetime risk for a disease, whereas environment determines whether or not that disease develops. However, recent research shows that early life influences — the intrauterine environment and infant diet — can also affect lifetime risk when it comes to obesity.

In one study, investigators divided females from a strain of lean rats into two groups: one group was fed a standard diet and remained lean, whereas the other group was fed a special diet and became obese. Then both groups of females were bred with lean males. The investigators discovered that offspring of the obese females tended to be heavier than offspring of the lean females, even though all offspring had the same genetic makeup and were fed the same diet.

Recently published research suggests that a related phenomenon occurs in humans. Jennie Brand-Miller and colleagues in Australia gave healthy pregnant women two diets with identical protein, carbohydrates, fats, and fiber but different glycemic indexes. Remarkably, infants whose mothers consumed a high-glycemic diet were ten times more likely to be large for gestational age than infants whose mothers consumed a low-glycemic diet.

In light of these findings, the best time for a mother to prevent obesity in her children may be before birth, and possibly before conception: by having a healthy body weight at the beginning of pregnancy and consuming a low-glycemic diet during pregnancy. Regarding factors in infancy, breastfeeding seems to decrease the risk of becoming obese later in childhood and adolescence, and the longer the duration of breastfeeding, the greater the protection appears to be.

Based on fifteen years of practice, I believe that low-glycemic eating offers an alternative to all this. I think of this approach not as a diet in the usual sense of the word, but rather as a *diet* according to its Greek definition: "a manner of living." Low-glycemic eating helps resolve the battle between mind and metabolism within your child and also helps prevent conflict between you and your child. Children get to eat as much as they want until they are satisfied, because low-glycemic eating is designed to control excessive hunger at its biological source. As Michael from chapter 2 said, "My tastes have almost completely changed . . . Things like nut butters and cottage cheese taste good to me now. They make me feel fuller."

4

GETTING PHYSICAL

Ten thousand years ago. The sun is rising over Mount Kilimanjaro as fourteen-year-old Jimiyu sets out on foot with other members of his tribe in search of food. For two days, they alternate walking, jogging, sprinting, and resting as they hunt down a wild antelope and bring it back to their camp. Jimiyu's younger sisters are equally active. They walk up to five miles a day to gather wild plants and carry pots of water. To celebrate successful hunting and gathering expeditions, the children walk fifteen miles with the rest of their tribe to a neighboring camp, where they spend hours dancing and playing games.

One thousand years ago. Animals have been domesticated and vegetables are grown and harvested. Jin, a twelve-year-old boy who lives in a farming village in China, does not have to hunt for his next meal. Instead, he helps plant and harvest rice and vegetables, which have become the staples of his family's diet. The work is challenging and forces him to walk, squat, and dig for most of the day.

One hundred years ago. Eight-year-old Guinevere lives in a European city, where her father runs a flower shop. After school, she helps her mother shop for food, walking to the fish market, fruit store, and vegetable stand and carrying home hefty bags of groceries. Guinevere walks wherever she goes, which on most days includes a park. There she runs, skips, and swings with her neighborhood friends. She spends weekends hiking with her family.

America today. Jim, seventeen years old, sits in front of a TV eating a double cheeseburger with a large serving of fries, washing them down with a two-liter cola purchased from the seat of his car at a drive-through. He changes channels from the couch by pressing a button on a remote control. For dinner he devours a pizza that was delivered to his doorstep, then sits down at his computer to do homework and surf the Internet. At 5 feet 8 inches tall, Jim weighs more than 220 pounds. He is easily winded after climbing a flight of stairs and suffers from joint pain in his ankles and knees when he walks more than a block.

Biologically, there's little difference between Jimiyu and Jim. Their bodies are both designed to bend, climb, crouch, run, sprint, squat, twist, walk, and move in dozens of different ways. Jim's world, however, has radically changed. Physical activity is no longer an essential part of day-to-day life. According to a Kaiser Family Foundation study of more than 2,000 kids throughout the United States, adolescents like Jim spend less than one and a half hours a day doing any type of physical activity. They spend six hours a day — more than forty hours a week — in sedentary pursuits, such as watching TV, playing video games, and working on the computer. Amazingly, ten- to sixteen-year-olds engage in vigorous activity for just twelve minutes a day on average, as reported by Richard Strauss of Robert Wood Johnson Medical School.

Never before has a generation of children been so sedentary. What are the physical and emotional consequences of this dramatic drop in physical activity? How will it affect our children's risks for conditions such as diabetes, heart disease, and osteoporosis? What about their

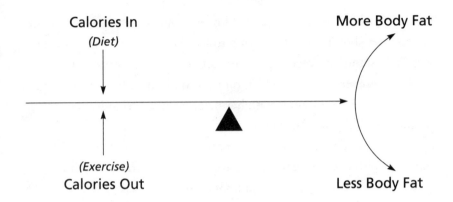

Figure 4.1 The Conventional View of Calorie Balance

self-esteem and mental health? Importantly, what can parents do to help their children become more physically active? To answer these questions, we'll take a fresh look at the science relating to physical activity, weight, and health. Then we'll present a six-point game plan to help transform even the most confirmed couch potato into an ardent action hero.

PE 101

You've heard it before: the only way to lose weight is to eat less and exercise more. Exercise tips the scale in favor of becoming thin; eating too much tips the scale in the opposite direction. According to this conventional view, diet and exercise are in competition and pushing in opposite directions (see Figure 4.1).

At first glance, the contest between diet and exercise seems depressingly unfair: jogging a full mile consumes only about 70 calories. So it would require a full marathon to burn off the 2,000 calories in just one supersize fast food meal. For this reason, weight loss efforts that focus on physical activity alone, without attention to diet, rarely produce significant results. Fortunately, the contest between diet and exercise is not as one-sided as it appears.

The Calorie Cavalry

When it comes to burning off calories, exercise has many allies, as shown in Figure 4.2. These include the following:

Growth: Children trying to lose weight have a huge advantage over adults: they're still growing. Growth and development consume a great deal of energy, especially during puberty. That's why, until very recently, it was so unusual to see an overweight teen. The good news is that all but the heaviest children can "grow" into their weight simply by slowing down their rate of weight gain. In general, one inch in height equates to about four or five pounds. So for an overweight child, maintaining weight unchanged for one year would, in effect, be the same as an adult losing ten or more pounds, depending on the child's age and growth rate.

Metabolic Rate: Metabolic rate is like the idle of a car when it sits in the driveway with the engine running. Even though the car is not moving, it still uses gasoline. Likewise, our bodies use energy constantly, even when we are not doing anything. Low thyroid hormone and some other medical problems can lower metabolic rate, and consequently cause weight gain, although these conditions account for at most 1 to 2 percent of all childhood obesity. Metabolic rate is also influenced by genes, which we can't control, and lifestyle, which we can.

Play: Long before treadmills, stationary bikes, stair-climbers, and even physical education classes, children had a secret strategy for staying active. It's called play. Play is the natural, spontaneous way that children amuse and occupy themselves. Many children easily expend more energy during play, because it is fun and engaging, than during structured activities such as organized sports. And as shown by Robert Whitaker and Hillary Burdette, a husband and wife research team in Philadelphia, play has benefits that extend far beyond weight control,

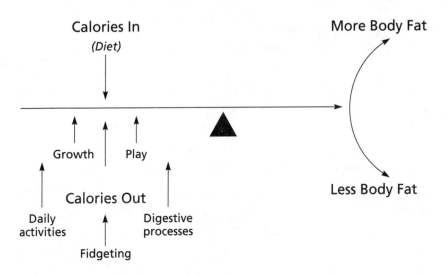

Figure 4.2 A Newer View of Calorie Balance

including development of cognitive abilities, improvement of social skills, and stress release.

NEAT: The term "non-exercise activity thermogenesis," or NEAT, describes the calories we use by movements other than intentional exercise. Ordinary activities such as walking around the house, standing, shifting positions in a chair, and even fidgeting use energy that can add up over time. To illustrate this point, researchers gathered a group of 20 "self-proclaimed couch potatoes" and measured body movements, including how often they stood, sat, and lay down, every half second for ten days. In all, the researchers collected about 25 million measurements related to posture and movement for each person. Half of the group was obese and the other half lean. The obese individuals, it turned out, sat for an average of 2 hours and 40 minutes longer than the lean individuals each day, whereas the lean individuals remained upright for 2 hours and 30 minutes longer than the obese individuals. The researchers concluded that if the obese individuals adopted the simple movement patterns of their lean counterparts, they could burn an additional 350 calories a day, theoretically equal to about thirty-five pounds of weight loss per year. What does this mean for your child? Even seemingly inconsequential activities can add up over the course of a day, a week, and a childhood.

Digestion: We even burn calories when we eat, digest, and absorb our food. In fact, the heat released by digestion may be a key "satiety signal," giving us that warm, satisfied feeling after a good meal and letting our brain know that we've had enough.

Exercise and its allies don't just operate independently; they can actually act synergistically to promote weight loss. For example, all forms of physical activity build muscle, and muscle is far more metabolically active than fat. So regular physical activity not only burns calories while we're doing it, but it also increases metabolic rate throughout the day, even while we're sleeping.

Activity and Diet: A Secret Alliance

They may seem like adversaries, but physical activity and diet quietly cooperate with each other to tip the scales in favor of weight gain or weight loss, depending on the situation. Let's look at some examples.

Diet can influence metabolic rate. Eating an adequate amount of protein helps build muscle, which, as we just saw, supports a fast metabolism. However, a low-glycemic diet may have similar benefits at any level of protein intake. To examine this point, we fed two groups of rats diets with equal amounts of protein, fats, and carbohydrates, differing only in glycemic index. At seven weeks, the rats on the high-glycemic diet started burning off fewer calories than those on the low-glycemic diet, and this gap increased progressively with time. The reason for this slow metabolism became obvious when we measured body composition. Although both groups of rats were kept at the same weight, the high–glycemic index animals had 70 percent more fat, with a corresponding decrease in lean tissue.

The kinds of food we eat may have special importance during weight loss, regardless of how much lean tissue we have. As described in chapter 3, we fed overweight and obese young adults two low-calorie diets, either low fat or low glycemic, as they lost 10 percent of their weight over about ten weeks. Even though both groups had the same amount of body fat and lean tissue throughout the study, metabolic rate remained 80 calories per day faster after weight loss in those on the low-glycemic diet than in those on the low-fat diet.

Diet can influence how many calories are burned after eating. It takes energy to digest and metabolize all types of food, but different types require varying amounts of energy to process: protein the most energy, fats the least, and carbohydrates, depending in part on their glycemic index, somewhere in between. Overall, the amount of energy expended during digestion is small — about 10 percent of our daily calorie intake — but these differences can add up over time.

Diet can influence physical activity level. Visualize just having eaten the following meal (just this once): a bacon double cheeseburger, large fries, a shake, and a package of chocolate chip cookies. Now how would you feel? Ready for a rousing game of soccer, a bracing swim, or the elliptical machine at the gym? How about a couch near a TV or, better yet, a bed? Those double servings of fast food can cause double trouble when it comes to body weight. Not only do we overconsume calories, but we're also not likely to burn them off anytime soon.

Similarly, consuming a high-glycemic snack of pretzels and juice might provide a quick energy boost but will soon leave us fatigued and less inclined to exercise for long as blood sugar quickly drops. When researchers gave 10 trained cyclists either a low- or a high-glycemic meal thirty minutes before beginning a vigorous ride, they found that those who consumed the low-glycemic meal had more stable blood sugar levels than those who consumed the high-glycemic meal, and they were able to bike 60 percent longer before reaching exhaustion. Several other studies of sports performance have reached the same conclusion.

**Physical activity can influence stress, mood, and mental health —
and consequently eating habits.** One of the most important benefits of
physical activity is how it makes us feel. Among 20,000 adolescent and
adult twins in the Netherlands, those who reported at least moderate
levels of exercise were less anxious, neurotic, and depressed and more
outgoing than non-exercisers. In England, nine- and ten-year-old children who exercised for fifteen minutes had more positive feelings and
fewer negative feelings, whereas the opposite happened after fifteen
minutes of watching a video. And researchers in Japan and Thailand
studied 49 young women, ages eighteen to twenty, with mild to moderate depression. Half were given an exercise program consisting of
five light jogging sessions each week, and the other half followed their
usual activities. After eight weeks, the jogging group showed an improvement in depressive symptoms, whereas the usual activities group
showed no improvement. Of particular interest, activity even influenced biological signs of stress, as levels of the stress hormones adrenaline (epinephrine) and cortisol were significantly reduced in the jogging group. (High cortisol levels increase appetite and cause storage of
fat around the belly.) Indeed, studies have shown that physical activity
triggers the release of endorphins and other "feel good" substances in
the brain. It stands to reason that when we feel good, and feel good
about ourselves, we are much more likely to eat well.

And there's one more way that physical activity can affect eating
habits. Ever tried to eat a bag of chips while swimming? How about
while watching TV or surfing the Internet? You get the point.

From Vicious Cycle to Victorious Cycle

From this perspective, Figure 4.1 and even Figure 4.2 are too simple.
In reality, diet and activity are more intimately linked. For many overweight children like Tamica, the situation is closer to Figure 4.3.

I first met Tamica when she was nine years old. Her mother,
Maxine, who was also quite heavy, said that lately Tamica had been

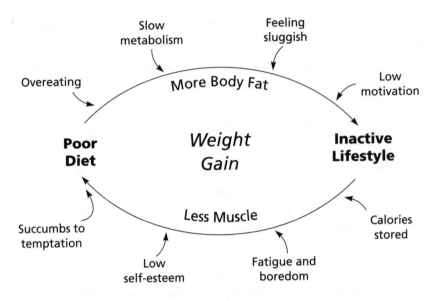

Figure 4.3 A Vicious Cycle

coming home from school in tears about her weight, especially upset that she could no longer fit into jeans. Recently outgrowing a size 16, Tamica instead had to wear stretch pants. Unfortunately, the family had limited social and financial support. Tamica's father was out of the picture entirely, and her grandmother was partially disabled. To make ends meet, Maxine often worked until early evening. With her mother away in the afternoon, Tamica stayed at home, watching TV and eating junk food. To deal with the stress of their lives, they ate out frequently and regularly treated themselves to ice cream.

Tamica continued to gain weight during her first four months in OWL. The more weight she gained, the worse she felt physically and emotionally. And the worse she felt, the harder it was for her to make even the smallest change in her eating and activity habits. Food and TV had become her only refuge: a vicious cycle.

The problem for Tamica, and for so many of us, is that vicious cycles have a momentum of their own. Once they get going, they tend to keep going. Slowing down and finally stopping the spin often requires

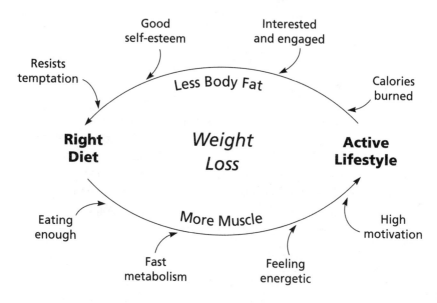

Figure 4.4 A Victorious Cycle

a concerted effort directed at several components of the cycle. In time, however, the direction of the spin can be reversed into a victorious cycle (see Figure 4.4).

I didn't see Tamica again in OWL for some time and had assumed that she'd given up. So I was happy to see her name on my list of patients one day about eight months after her initial appointment. When she and her mother arrived, I was surprised: both were notably thinner, and Tamica seemed happier than I had ever seen her. I asked them what happened.

Maxine told me that one day, about three months earlier, she decided it was time to get rid of the extra weight she had carried from her second pregnancy the year before. She stopped bringing junk food into her home. Instead of eating out or taking out most nights, Maxine made a quick but nutritious family dinner. And she began going for evening walks with Tamica on a regular basis. Because of Maxine's busy schedule, this required a considerable amount of planning and coordination with the grandmother, who lived nearby and helped out.

SLEEP ON IT

❖ Recent studies have identified sleep deprivation as a major risk factor for excessive weight gain in both adults and children. In one study involving five- and six-year-olds, those sleeping less than ten hours on weekdays were twice as likely to be overweight compared to those sleeping more than eleven and a half hours. Sleep deprivation seems to upset the normal daily rhythm of hormone production, creating a biological tendency to store fat. And without adequate sleep, it can be difficult to find the energy and motivation to eat right and be active. So when it comes to losing weight, remember that what we do at night may be just as important as what we do during the day.

At first Tamica went along with these changes kicking and screaming, "throwing a fit" when Maxine tried to limit her portion sizes. Within a few weeks, however, Tamica was amazed to discover that she could once again fit into her size 16 jeans. Soon she stopped resisting the changes and actually joined her mother's weight loss efforts. She signed up for an afterschool fitness program and cut back on her TV time. In addition, Tamica began paying attention to what and how much she ate. She discovered that, in time, "her stomach shrank," and she would feel satisfied with less food.

Tamica admits that she "still has a sweet tooth." But now, instead of always giving in to temptation, she redirects her attention to two favorite pursuits, drawing and writing. Since Tamica feels healthier and more confident, making the right choices has become much easier. And she is thrilled about an upcoming shopping trip: it seems that her size 16 pants are rapidly becoming too big. A victorious cycle has started to spin.

Immobilized by Aliens

Imagine that aliens have taken over Earth. To keep us under their control, they implant a strange and powerful device in our homes. This device hypnotizes us into a trancelike state in which our metabolism slows down as much as or more than it does while we're sleeping. Even worse, the device tricks us into eating massive amounts of extremely high-calorie, low-quality foods. Soon we grow too heavy and unfit to resist the alien invasion; eventually we develop life-threatening diseases. We lose on average ten years of life per person, a figure that will rise rapidly if nothing is done to stop the invasion.

OK, the aliens in this story were made up, but the effects of that mind control device — what we call TV — were not. Each day, Americans watch more than half a billion hours of TV, amounting to almost ten years per person throughout his or her life. And if we consider how TV contributes to obesity, heart disease, diabetes, and a range of other life-shortening medical conditions, the amount of time we sacrifice to it may be even greater.

Of the many environmental factors that contribute to excessive weight gain in kids, TV may be the most influential. In a landmark study in 1996, Steven Gortmaker and colleagues at Harvard School of Public Health examined a nationally representative group of 750 children ages ten to fifteen years. They found that the risk of becoming overweight was an astounding fivefold greater among children watching TV five hours or more each day compared to those watching two hours or less. Based on these data, the authors calculated that 60 percent or more of all childhood overweight might be attributable to excessive TV viewing. A similar conclusion was reached by researchers at the University of Michigan. Studying 1,000 three-year-olds around the country, they found that watching two or more hours of TV per day increased the risk of becoming overweight by threefold. And in a third study, involving adolescents ages twelve to seventeen, researchers at the University of Kansas found that body mass index increased almost one unit (about six pounds) for every additional hour of TV viewing per day. The reason for this dramatic effect is that TV powerfully influences both sides of the body weight equation: more calories go in, and fewer are burned off.

Certainly, TV takes time away from active pursuits such as organized sports, playing, or even walking, which all use energy. Worse, children's metabolism may plummet to extraordinarily low levels when they watch TV. Robert Klesges and colleagues in Memphis measured the metabolic rate of 15 overweight and 16 normal weight girls ages eight to twelve years. The researchers took two different measurements of metabolism, one while the girls were at rest and the other while they watched TV. They found that both the overweight and normal weight girls' metabolic rates were on average more than 200 calories per day lower while watching TV. In terms of weight control, they would probably have been better off asleep.

A second way that TV leads to weight gain is through the mouth, a point that was graphically demonstrated in a novel video diary project involving OWL. Together with Michael Rich, a colleague at Children's Hospital Boston, we gave video cameras to some of our patients and simply asked them to document their lives. Rich's work has shown that video diaries can give medical providers unique insights into their patients' lives. In addition, children often become much more conscious of unhealthful behaviors when they view themselves from this perspective.

The scenes that came back astonished everyone, including the kids. Our patients not only spent much of their free time watching TV but also displayed extreme eating behaviors in front of the TV. One teenager came into the room with a family-size bag of popcorn, turned on the TV, and, in robotlike fashion, brought fistful after fistful of food to his mouth. Another teen sat with a plate of hot dogs, consuming each in one or two bites, barely chewing, all the while staring vacantly at the TV.

These videos revealed that the food children consume while

watching TV may affect their calorie balance far more than just being sedentary does. This is just what Len Epstein, a renowned pediatric psychologist at the University of Buffalo, found. Epstein's team performed a nine-week study with 13 children ages eight to twelve years and their families. During the initial three-week phase, the children went about life, eating and exercising according to their usual habits. During the next two 3-week phases, the families were told to either increase or decrease their sedentary activities (principally watching TV and videos, playing video games, and using the computer) but not to make any changes in their diets. The children's activity levels were determined by diaries and accelerometers (devices that measure movement), and diets were assessed by telephone interviews. The researchers found that when the children became more sedentary, their energy balance went up by 350 calories per day. But only a small part of this change, 100 calories per day, was due to decreased physical activity; most of it, 250 calories per day, was from increased food intake. And virtually all of the sedentary eating took place while they were watching TV, not playing video games or using the computer.

Tom Robinson at Stanford University came to a similar conclusion after providing an eighteen-lesson classroom curriculum to third- and fourth-grade students at an elementary school in San Jose, California. The curriculum was designed to reduce the use of TV, videotapes, and video games. After six months, Robinson found that body weight was lower among these children — by half a BMI unit, or about three pounds — compared to other students at a nearby elementary school who didn't receive the curriculum. Of particular interest, there was no difference between the two groups of students in level of moderate to vigorous physical activity or level of fitness. The main difference between the groups: fewer meals in front of the TV for those participating in the curriculum.

Of special concern is the effect of TV on the youngest children. Leann Birch at Pennsylvania State University examined the lunchtime eating habits of 24 preschool children one day while they were watching a TV cartoon and another day without TV. Among the children who frequently ate in front of the TV at home, calorie consumption went up by one-third on the day the cartoon was shown. The finding raises the possibility that regular TV viewing during meals might desensitize young children to normal satiety signals — the way that the body tells us when it's had enough. If a young child learns to ignore these signals, what might happen later in life?

Possibly the most important reason TV contributes to obesity relates to its effects on children not just while they're watching but also throughout the day, and perhaps throughout life. It is the primary reason for TV's existence in the first place: advertising. Generally, more money is spent on the commercials shown during a TV show than on creating the show itself, totaling many billions of dollars per year. Each day, a typical child sees dozens of food ads — almost exclusively for fast food, junk food, and sugar-sweetened drinks.

A particularly worrisome development is that the line once separating TV shows and commercials has been blurred beyond recognition. Popular TV characters such as SpongeBob and Scooby-Doo entertain kids during the program and then sell sugary cereals, macaroni and cheese, and the like during commercials. Ronald McDonald has become one of the most recognizable characters among American children, second only to Santa Claus. Even if you, as a parent, gave a positive nutritional message to your child at every meal, you'd be undermined by commercials at a rate of 10 to 1. Indeed, the evidence chain linking TV viewing to obesity by way of overall diet is now solid enough to satisfy even the most cautious district attorney. Studies clearly show that when children see food ads:

- They are more likely to ask (or, more accurately, nag) their parents to buy the advertised products.
- Their parents are more likely to purchase those products.
- They are more likely to consume the advertised products.
- They are less likely to eat healthful foods, such as fruits and vegetables.
- Their calorie intake goes up.

In her powerful book *Food Politics,* Marion Nestle shows how marketing firms actually conduct studies to determine the number of times a child has to nag a parent for a product before the parent caves in and buys it. The firms call this phenomenon the "nag factor." Manipulating children through seductive advertising designed by child psychologists on their payrolls, these companies bombard children with images, gifts, slogans, and jingles that create cravings and lead to peer pressure, which in turn lead children to demand and eat their products.

A recent study by Steven Gortmaker and Jean Wiecha at Harvard, in which I participated, illustrates the insidious effects of advertising on diet quality. We examined the eating and TV viewing patterns of 500 middle school children in Cambridge, Massachusetts, over a two-year period. We found that for every additional hour of TV viewing, children consumed an extra 167 calories, almost entirely from sugar-sweetened beverages, salty snacks, fried potatoes, sweet baked snacks, candy, and fast food — no coincidence the foods most commonly advertised on TV.

Most concerning of all is that TV may affect children long into the future. Researchers in New Zealand examined 1,000 individuals from birth through young adulthood. They found that TV viewing during childhood was associated with increased body weight, higher cholesterol, and lower cardiopulmonary fitness at age twenty-six. Indeed, childhood TV viewing habits were more strongly related to these risk factors than adult viewing habits. In other words, the lifestyle patterns taught by TV to children may "program" them for a lifetime of obesity and poor health.

Stretching Beyond Weight Loss

As your child begins to increase physical activity and reduce TV time, she will start to build muscle and reduce fat. Her self-esteem will improve, and so will her eating habits. These in turn will help her become even more active. But the benefits of physical activity extend well beyond weight loss. Regular physical activity also reduces the risks for a number of important medical problems, even without losing a pound.

Diabetes: The single most important cause of diabetes is excessive body weight. Physical activity helps prevent diabetes at any body weight by improving the sensitivity of our tissues to the hormone insulin. Fifty-nine overweight middle school children in rural Wisconsin were given either a fitness-oriented gym class or the standard gym class for an academic year. At the end of the program, neither group had lost any weight, but the fitness group showed a decrease in insulin level, whereas the standard gym group showed an increase.

Heart Disease: Physical activity has beneficial effects on a host of traditional and newly discovered heart disease risk factors, including high blood pressure, high cholesterol, chronic inflammation, and abnormal blood-clotting tendency. These conditions don't just affect older adults; many have been identified in overweight children as young as five years of age. A study of overweight children and adolescents from Minnesota showed that some of these abnormalities can be improved in as little as eight weeks of a stationary cycling program.

Osteoporosis: Thinning bones may be something you associate with old age, but its roots can stretch back to childhood. Among a group of Caucasian girls, physical activity before puberty was related to bone thickness in late adolescence.

WARNING: ADOLESCENCE MAY BE HAZARDOUS TO YOUR DAUGHTER'S HEALTH

❖ At no time in a girl's life does she accumulate more body fat than during adolescence. This is in part a biological necessity, since females reaching reproductive age need a critical amount of fat to support a successful pregnancy. But for many girls, excessive weight gain is less about biology and more about behavior. Girls are more likely than boys to abandon physical activity as they enter their teens. This drop in physical activity, perhaps more than any change in eating habits, may be the problem.

Consider the findings of a study that tracked the physical activities — including organized sports, recreational activities, and walking — of more than 2,200 black and white girls beginning at age ten in three U.S. cities. After ten years, the group as a whole was doing 83 percent less activity than when they started. By the time the girls were sixteen or seventeen years old, 56 percent of black girls and 31 percent of white girls said they did absolutely no physical activity outside of gym class. Not surprisingly, this sharp drop-off in physical activity resulted in excessive weight gain. The girls who reported being inactive gained an average of ten to fifteen pounds more than their active friends, even though there was little difference in the number of calories the two groups consumed.

❖ Sadly, teenage girls are especially susceptible to body image issues and eating disorders such as binge eating and bulimia nervosa (binging and purging), and TV only adds fuel to the fire. As summarized by William Dietz back in 1990, "the [infrequent depiction] of obesity among televised characters, combined with the frequent food-related references that are contained in both commercials and programming, may promote unrealistic conclusions regarding eating and body weight. Television reflects a cultural contradiction by promoting food consumption and leanness. In this context, [television may cause] bulimia . . . because only bulimics can eat everything they wish and remain thin."

The Game Plan

Now that you're warmed up, let's get moving with a six-point game plan designed to take weight control into high gear.

1. **Deprogram Your Child.** Get rid of the TV and cancel the cable subscription. OK, this might be a bit extreme. Instead, how about offering these ground rules.
   - Limit TV viewing to two hours a day (good), one hour a day (better), or one-half hour a day (best).
   - Take the TV out of your child's bedroom and avoid watching during meals.
   - Encourage your child to watch public TV stations instead of commercial stations. Not only is the quality of programming higher, but these stations also tend not to run food advertisements.
   - Keep a written log of viewing habits. Whenever family members (including parents) turn on the TV, have them record what show(s) they watched and for how long. Review these logs on a weekly basis with the whole family.
   - Make TV viewing dependent on physical activity, such as walking on a treadmill or riding a stationary bike placed in front of the set. Linking TV viewing to physical activity neutralizes two of the three ways that TV contributes to obesity: decreased calorie expenditure and mindless eating while watching (though viewers are still vulnerable to the influence of food ads).
2. **Play.** When it comes to physical activity, children, especially before puberty, aren't mini adults. Metabolically, children aren't capable of the sustained endurance activities — such as jogging or working out at the gym — that adults so commonly equate with exercise. Mentally, they don't naturally maintain an intense focus on one activity for long. For these reasons, play is the perfect solution. Plus, it's fun. So try not even to use the "e" word.

When four-year-old Alison returned home from a birthday party at a sports center — her smiling face flushed from two hours of running, jumping, and climbing with friends — her mother commented that she must have gotten a lot of exercise. Alison looked perplexed. "No, Mommy, we didn't exercise," she insisted. "We just played!"

First and foremost, provide your child with opportunities to be in nature: parks, playgrounds, a meadow, the mountains, or just the backyard. Being outdoors naturally inspires us to be active. Give your child access to age-appropriate toys that encourage activity: a ball, a Frisbee, a shovel and pail, a jump rope, roller skates (with protective gear), or a bike (with a helmet). For younger children, find ways for them to play with other children in a safe setting. Many older children and adolescents enjoy the challenge of sports, although some who are very overweight prefer noncompetitive group activities such as swimming or yoga. Dancing can be a great option for kids of all ages, including boys. It's also important to spend as much active time as possible together as a family. An afternoon at the beach or a stroll after dinner are two options.

The Lowell family has learned how to turn family time into a physical affair. With two adolescent girls, two working parents, and dozens of social, professional, and community-related commitments to juggle, the family has to work to spend time together. In the past, family time usually meant going out to dinner and to a movie, where they shared a large bucket of buttered popcorn, passing it back and forth until every kernel was gone. But when thirteen-year-old Leslie joined the OWL Program, the Lowells decided to find healthier ways to be together. Now, on some nights, instead of going out, they take long walks near their home, and on weekends they take hikes. Today, the Lowells are looking forward to their second annual family camping trip. And when they do see a movie, they pass up the popcorn and sneak in their own snacks of grapes and apples.

TURNING THE TABLES:
TECHNOLOGY THAT MOVES

❖ Some kids have managed to turn their PlayStation, GameCube, or Xbox — technology not typically used for physical activities — into a virtual gym. In Dance Dance Revolution (DDR), flashing arrows direct players to move their feet according to a pattern designated on a mat, all to the beat of a song. Similar games include MC Groovz, Dance Drum, Dance Pad, Dance Factory, and Flow: Urban Dance Uprising. "You're not thinking of it like exercise," Leslie said, describing dance competitions she now has at home with her younger sister. "With DDR, you're tired, but you're happy about it. You're just having fun."

3. **Easy Does It.** Some people derive great enjoyment from long runs, arduous hikes, competitive sports, or intense workouts at the gym. For the less athletic among us, these activities can seem intimidating. And for overweight kids, vigorous endeavors can be unattainable and even unsafe, at least at first. Fortunately, light to moderate physical activity — if made a regular part of our lifestyles — is all that we need to increase self-confidence, improve fitness, and promote weight loss. To demonstrate this point, researchers studied the metabolism of obese preteenage boys as they walked at different speeds. They found that the highest rate of fat burning was achieved when the boys walked at a leisurely pace of less than three miles per hour; walking faster didn't increase the rate of fat burning. The bottom line is that all kinds of physical activity are beneficial.

So let's liberate ourselves and our kids from the boot camp mentality of exercise. A physically active lifestyle isn't just for jocks, and it doesn't have to hurt.

SOTHERN COMFORT

❖ Melinda Sothern of Louisiana State University is an expert in childhood fitness and coauthor of *Trim Kids*. Here are her eight easy tips for making physical activity fun.

1. Encourage children to do something active and fun when they get home from school, before doing their homework, such as riding a bike, walking the dog, skating, dancing to their favorite songs, or playing tag outside. Afterward, they'll concentrate better on their studies.

2. Create a physical activity center with safe, indoor active toys and games in a corner of the family room. Call it an imagination station.

3. Discourage TV and computer time by turning on the stereo when you get home. Teach your children to cha-cha, tango, or waltz, or let them teach you the latest dance craze.

4. Encourage your children to dance or stretch during TV commercials.

5. Give physically active choices: clean your room or walk the dog; help wash the car or dance in your room; help rake leaves or go for a bike ride.

6. Young children are best suited for short bursts of intermittent active play — such as tag — so be careful not to impose adult exercise goals, programs, or equipment on them.

7. Enroll your children in an activity that encourages movement, such as organized sports, dance, martial arts, swimming, tennis, or gymnastics, once per week. This will encourage friendships with other physically active children.

8. Reserve at least one day each weekend dedicated to fun family fitness activities. Participate in activities the entire family can enjoy together. Go for a family bike ride, hike, or fly kites.

A SCHOOL THAT ROCKS

❖ If there's one place where kids are often admonished to "sit still and be quiet," it's the classroom. But researcher James Levine from the Mayo Clinic is challenging the long-standing belief that kids need to remain motionless as they learn. His experimental classroom is set up so that its fourth- and fifth-grade students can move and fidget while listening to their teacher give the daily lesson. Levine replaced standard desk and chair sets with adjustable podiums that allow kids to stand or kneel. Kids can also bounce or balance on exercise balls. To measure whether his experiment is having an impact, students wear sensors that measure muscle movements. According to Levine, "The sensors indeed demonstrate that when you give kids the opportunity to move, they will do so." While Levine doesn't think that his classroom is the answer to the childhood obesity epidemic, he is betting that it will help.

4. **Get NEAT!** Even for those of us who regularly set aside time for structured physical activity, what happens during those twenty, forty, or sixty minutes each day probably matters less than what happens during the rest of the day. As discussed earlier in this chapter, non-exercise activity thermogenesis (NEAT) can amount to many hundreds of calories each day, depending on what we do when we're *not* intending to exercise. These forms of "stealth" physical activity — easy to incorporate without our kids even realizing it — can play a major role in preventing weight gain, and maintaining weight loss, if done on a regular basis.

   • Walk rather than drive wherever and whenever possible.
   • Take the stairs instead of the elevator.
   • Ask your child to help out with household chores that require physical activity, such as gardening or sweeping up (or washing dishes, if you can manage it).

THE "SPORTS-ADE" CHARADE

❖ In the past few years, so-called sports drinks — the ones whose names end in "ade" — have been heavily marketed as healthful alternatives to traditional soft drinks. True, they have a few added minerals, but this difference is meaningless in all but the most extreme athletic scenarios. In most cases, when children consume these drinks regularly, they can easily take in more calories than they burn off.

- Encourage your child to take five-minute "stand and stretch" breaks every thirty minutes when sedentary (such as with TV, computer, or homework).
- Even fidgeting can burn off calories that add up over time. Before you tell your squirming child to sit still, think again!

5. **Walk the Walk.** Sometimes parents don't do things that benefit their health (such as quitting smoking) until they realize that their children will also benefit (from less exposure to secondhand smoke). Guess what? When parents get active, it's not only good for them, it's also good for the kids. A number of studies have shown that physical activity habits are learned from the family. For example, researchers in France found that adolescents were almost twice as likely to participate in structured physical activities outside school if both parents practiced a sport. Conversely, teenage boys were twice as likely to be highly inactive if both parents watched TV more than two hours each day. Set a positive example by making physical activity a priority for yourself. If your children see you make time for it, they will, too. Your efforts will pay off for years to come, as active kids tend to stay active for life.

6. **Food + Action = Success.** Despite its many benefits, physical activity alone rarely results in dramatic short-term weight loss. For a typical child, an increase in moderately vigorous activity of one

hour each day will produce less than a two-pound weight loss in a month. Although these pounds will add up over many months or years, the greatest benefits are achieved when the muscles and the mouth work together, as shown in Figure 4.4. To help your child get the most from being active, fuel her body with a balanced, low-glycemic diet.

Cooling Down and Looking Ahead

We may not be able to return to the days of Jimiyu, Jin, or even Guinevere, when physical activity was an integral part of day-to-day life. But we can support our children to have an active lifestyle.

Sometimes we think that we — and our children — don't have time to get physical in our busy, modern world. But by encouraging our children to engage in physical activity, we can actually improve the quality of their lives overall. Take thirteen-year-old Leslie, whom we met earlier in this chapter. Leslie has been on the honor roll throughout middle school and always makes homework her top priority. Since Leslie enjoys swimming, her mother suggested that she join the swim team as a way of pursuing her weight loss goal. Leslie agreed to do this but was quite concerned that her grades would suffer if she took time away from her studies. "She worries about her homework a lot, and that almost gets in her way," said her mother, who initially had to "drag" Leslie to swim practice. But after a while, Leslie began noticing that swimming had other benefits besides weight loss.

"She realizes now that when she exercises and gets all of this stress out first, she can sit down and focus and get her homework done quicker," her mother said.

Leslie agreed, noting, "I never wanted to admit it, but when I go to swimming, I actually feel a lot better, and I can focus more on what I have to do."

Looking at life from this perspective, do we have time *not* to get active?

5

IT'S THE THOUGHT
THAT COUNTS

In chapter 2, we saw why it's so important for everyone, especially children, to maintain a healthy weight. In chapters 3 and 4, we looked at novel approaches to nutrition and physical activity that work with our basic biological makeup. Of course, the world's best diet and activity plan won't work if people don't follow it. That's where psychology — how we think about ourselves and our world — comes into play.

I've rarely met an overweight child who doesn't want to be thin. However, most don't show up in my office brimming with enthusiasm and eager to embrace a weight loss program. Sometimes, as with Jared in chapter 2, resistance can be a form of rebellion relating to conflict at home. In such cases, effective parenting strategies are needed (see chapter 6). More frequently, however, resistance to weight loss is caused by negative thoughts and self-defeating beliefs — basic misperceptions that propagate themselves and immobilize us. We may believe that we will never lose weight no matter how hard we try, or that we deserve to be overweight because we're lazy or bad at sports. Fortunately, there are tools that allow us to shift our thought patterns and re-create our reality in profound ways, freeing us from this paralysis.

There are many different psychological theories for helping people change attitudes and behavior. In my experience, no one theory has all the answers for everyone. For this reason, we use a combination of tools in the OWL Program, including the following:

There's No Comparison

All too often we decide how we feel by comparing ourselves to others. An 85 on a test could make you feel pretty smart if a friend got a 75, but how would you feel if your friend scored a 95? Probably not so good. Girls are especially susceptible to this pattern of thinking, constantly comparing their bodies to others. This psychologically unhealthy practice is made far worse by the media, which present unrealistic images of female beauty. Fashion models, selected for extraordinary appearance, have their looks further exaggerated by makeup and lighting. More perversely, their images are often altered electronically to make their legs look extremely long or their hips unnaturally narrow, so that girls are ultimately comparing themselves to something that doesn't even exist. This is a recipe for self-contempt, depression, eating disorders, and giving up. A girl comes to understand that she'll never look like Kate Moss, so why even bother eating right and getting active? This self-defeating attitude, which stems from the tendency to judge oneself against others, leads to escalating weight and plummeting self-esteem: another vicious cycle.

In one study, researchers documented the harmful effects of negative social comparisons among 1,500 male and female adolescents in Nova Scotia. They found that exposure to idealized body images in the media, and the tendency to compare oneself to these images, predicted poor self-esteem, dissatisfaction with one's body, and unhealthy dieting practices. For boys, they also predicted the use of steroids to build muscle mass.

The ultimate solution is to stop the comparisons and realize that our self-worth has nothing to do with how we look. Each of us has a unique, special nature: let's honor and respect ourselves just as we are and not collaborate with the powerful commercial interests that would have us believe we must look a certain way. Accepting ourselves is not just the foundation of happiness; it is a vital prerequisite to change.

Action Plan:
Communicate with your child using the three Rs.

1. Reassurance: Counter peer pressure and media influences by consistently assuring your child that she is lovable and loved just as she is. Any discussion of body weight or any plan to begin a weight loss program should focus on objective benefits, such as feeling better, being able to participate in sports, and avoiding future health problems. (You may also suggest, gently, that losing weight might reduce teasing.) Reiterate that losing weight, or not, has nothing whatsoever to do with how much you love and value your child.

2. Reality testing: Emphasize that everyone has unique gifts and challenges. Discuss your child's strengths. Point out the difficulties you had to deal with as a child, or perhaps even deal with now. Tell her that staying thin is hard for almost everyone today. Three out of four adults and many children are struggling with weight just as she is. It's not her fault.

3. Reverse comparisons: For a child who can't think of anything good about herself, it's OK to find ways in which she compares favorably to others. Focus on inner qualities rather than physical attributes. For instance, point out that just being able to discuss weight issues honestly puts her in a very special category. Unlike so many others, she's beginning to take positive steps to address her weight problem. Too often, overweight children are highly skilled at comparing themselves physically to others while overlooking internal qualities such as kindness, generosity, and intelligence.

"WITH FRIENDS LIKE THESE . . ."
— A CONVERSATION TO HAVE WITH
YOUR DAUGHTER

❖ Weight is an issue that affects people in many different ways. You might consider addressing this issue with your daughter as follows.

"When you start to lose weight, not everyone is going to be as happy for you as we are. Sometimes a friend might feel threatened. Maybe your efforts are causing her to examine her own weight issues, and this is painful for her. Maybe she envies your drive and motivation and wishes she could be more like you. At times, she may even try to undermine your efforts by inviting you out for pizza or telling you that you're no longer fun to be around. If this happens, recognize that you have done nothing wrong. Develop strategies for getting out of sticky situations gracefully. If you know a group of friends is going out for pizza, have a satisfying snack beforehand. Then have one piece of pizza, a salad, and a no-calorie drink. If you're having trouble dealing with these types of friends, discuss your feelings with us."

Chain Reaction

Eating is sometimes at the end of a long chain of events that has nothing to do with hunger. Consider this example.

- Your daughter has a fight with her best friend.
- She leaves school feeling angry that her friend would treat her so badly.
- When she gets home, she's in a bad mood. She goes into her room, closes the door, and turns on the TV.
- A commercial for a sugary cereal comes on.

- She thinks about eating something sweet.
- She remembers the fight and grows increasingly angry, thinking she is better off without friends that treat her like that.
- She sees another commercial, this time for a chocolate cookie.
- She realizes that she didn't have her snack of fruit and cheese after school because she was so mad.
- She leaves her room, heads for the kitchen, and grabs a box of cereal.
- She pours some into a bowl and eats it quickly. The cereal tastes sweet as it practically melts on her tongue, providing a momentary distraction and emotional relief.
- After finishing the first bowl of cereal, she remembers how angry she is with her friend, then pours herself another bowl.
- She finishes the second bowl, then feels guilty about the splurge.
- She thinks that she's a failure and that she'll always be fat. She blames herself for the fight with her friend and feels sad.
- She finishes the entire box of cereal.

In one study, researchers found that obese women who binged regularly did so to cover up anger or sadness. After the binge, they felt guilty, but to them this emotion was preferable to feeling sad or angry. Trading one negative emotion for a more desirable negative emotion was the end result of a long chain reaction. If you suspect that your child eats out of anger, sadness, anxiety, or any other feeling, you can help him find alternative coping strategies for dealing with these negative emotions.

Action Plan:
- Together with your child, think of three situations in which each of you engages in emotional eating.
- For each of these situations, come up with one thing you can do to break the chain of events.
- Write these strategies down and post them on your refrigerator.

All or Nothing

Did you ever eat a whole pie because you thought you'd blown your diet with the first piece? Did you ever abandon an exercise program because you missed a few days? All-or-nothing thinking can turn a minor slip into a full-scale disaster. Eating one piece of pie doesn't mean you've failed and should give up your weight loss plan. As Yale's Kelly Brownell says, "Weight loss is like a game of Chutes and Ladders: sometimes you do well, sometimes you have a setback, but you'll get there eventually." You don't have to be perfect; no one is. The people who are successful at losing weight are those who can learn from the inevitable setbacks and continue on.

Sometimes all-or-nothing thinkers get in trouble after impressive initial accomplishments. They expect constant progress, but progress is rarely constant. Take fifteen-year-old Leticia, who began the OWL Program like a racehorse out of the gate. When she first came to see us, she weighed 250 pounds and had type 2 diabetes. Over the next few months, she was able to implement key dietary changes, including cutting back on juice, eating more fruits and vegetables, and limiting portion sizes of high-calorie foods. She started walking thirty minutes each day and even wore a pedometer to track her progress. In less than a year, Leticia's BMI decreased by four units, the equivalent of twenty-four pounds — a truly wonderful achievement.

But then something changed. Frequently, the first few extra pounds come off more easily than the last few. As Leticia's rate of weight loss slowed, she became discouraged and fell back into her old habits. She began skipping breakfast again and eating large amounts of processed snack foods. And she gave up her daily walk. Not surprisingly, she regained much of the weight she'd lost. She even stopped taking her diabetes medication, no longer seeing any point in controlling her disease. Fortunately, Leticia continued to work with OWL psychologists on a regular basis. Today, Leticia has recommitted herself to eating well and being active, and she is working to shift her thinking patterns to ones that are more flexible — and more forgiving.

Children can be their own worst enemies with all-or-nothing thinking, although parents also can fall into this trap. Twelve-year-old Aaron was enthusiastic about getting healthier when he first came to OWL. At the end of his initial consultation, he declared his intentions to cut back on his usual seven hours of TV and video a day and to trade in sugary cereals, cookies, and chicken nuggets for more natural, whole foods. To support Aaron, his mother agreed to stock the house with plenty of fresh fruits and vegetables and reduced-fat dairy products. But when they returned to OWL the following month, his mother felt frustrated. She had made a consistent effort to buy fresh produce, but some of it had ended up in the garbage. She said that unless Aaron ate each and every healthy food she purchased, she would no longer support his participation in OWL. This example of all-or-nothing thinking risked undermining the meaningful progress that Aaron had made.

Action Plan:
- Together with your child, identify three ways that each of you falls into the trap of all-or-nothing thinking. For example: "If I have one piece of pie, the day is ruined, and it no longer matters what I eat."
- Come up with three statements that counter this error in thinking. For example: "Having one piece of pie doesn't undo all of my other weight loss efforts. I can get right back on track."
- Repeat these statements to yourself next time you find yourself engaged in unhelpful thought patterns.

One Step at a Time

The Chinese philosopher Lao Tzu was probably not thinking about weight loss when he wrote, "A journey of a thousand miles begins with a single step." Nonetheless, the proverb might be useful when looking to lose weight, which can seem overwhelming at the start. Instead of becoming paralyzed by the length of the journey, focus on all of the small things you can do that will eventually get you where you want to go. Walking up a flight of stairs or saying no to a sugary dessert one night may not seem like much, but each step brings you closer to your weight loss goal.

Action Plan:
- Together with your child, write down one thing that each of you can do right now, today or this week, to help you both achieve or maintain a healthy body weight.
- Commit to doing it.

Out of Sight, Out of Mind

In 1997, I conducted my first research study of how food affects appetite. My colleagues and I gave overweight teenage boys meals with identical calories but different glycemic indexes. After the meals, we instructed the teenagers to let us know when they became very hungry, and we would provide them with a large snack platter. Based on when and how many snacks were consumed, we could determine how filling the meals had been. We kept participants in separate rooms so that they wouldn't influence each other's eating habits.

Initially, everything proceeded perfectly. As we conducted the study, first one, then another participant would request a snack platter. However, one day, a study nurse called me, concerned that all three participants were requesting snacks at exactly the same time. I hurried to the research unit and immediately noticed a strong and familiar smell. Apparently, the parent of a child not involved in the study had purchased buttered popcorn and heated it up in a nearby microwave, making the research unit smell like a movie theater. The smell made everyone, nurses and patients alike, hungry.

CIAO, NUTELLA

❖ Leslie will never forget the day her family emptied their kitchen of all unhealthy foods. By the time they had finished, everyone in the family had said goodbye to something — her younger sister to her ramen noodles ("I was really, really mad," she said) and her mother to her beloved Nutella, a chocolate breakfast spread she used on toast. Having grown up in Europe, her mother considered Nutella a dietary staple. "We even carried it in our suitcase when we went on vacation," she recalled.

After getting over the initial shock of seeing four laundry baskets filled with high-calorie drinks, sugary cereals, potato chips, and cookies, the family came to see the exercise as a necessary step toward a healthier lifestyle. To Leslie, knowing that she would no longer have to battle dietary temptations at night was a huge relief. "I definitely thought that when we got everything out of the house, there was actually hope that I would lose weight," she said.

The family continues to keep junk food out of their home. In her first two months with OWL, Leslie's BMI decreased by a full unit (six pounds). Her sister has learned to get along without ramen noodles, and her mother now eats her toast — whole wheat — with peanut butter. Today, most of the family's food resides in the refrigerator, not the pantry.

That event could have spelled ruin for the study. Fortunately, we had enough participants to see an overall effect of glycemic index on appetite despite the popcorn debacle. But this story highlights one of the greatest challenges for people trying to lose weight: appetite and the desire to eat are strongly influenced by our environment. All of us, and especially children, are surrounded by an enormous variety of visually appealing, pleasant-smelling, and tasty high-calorie foods. Many of these foods have been designed to override our bodies' natural appetite-regulating systems by combining sugar, fat, and salt in high concentrations with chemicals that artificially enhance taste. Sooner or later, our motivation wavers just a bit, and we succumb to temptation. As we saw in chapter 3, eating the right way helps us feel full longer, which in turn helps us resist temptation. But why subject ourselves to unhealthful temptations at all, especially at home?

The tendency to eat simply because food is present was demonstrated in a study by Brian Wansink and colleagues at Cornell University involving 40 adult secretaries. Over a four-week period, the researchers placed chocolate candies in either clear or opaque bowls located either next to or six feet away from the secretaries' desks. After work hours, the researchers refilled the bowls and tallied how many candies had been eaten that day. The bowls were rotated so that each secretary spent an equal amount of time with the clear and opaque bowls, as well as next to the candy and six feet away from it.

Not surprisingly, the secretaries ate an extra 2.2 pieces of candy a day when the chocolate was visible through the clear bowl, and an extra 1.8 pieces when the bowl sat next to their desks. The take-home message for your child is that easy availability of junk food can trigger overeating.

Action Plan:
Turn your home into a "nutritional safe zone." Clean out cupboards and purge the pantry of all foods that are high in sugar and calories and short on nutrients and fiber. Replace them with healthy alternatives. Make this a family affair. (See Week 1 of the 9-Week Program in chapter 7.)

What's in a Name?

Quite a bit, it turns out. Take this example from politics. For many years, Americans widely supported the estate tax as a fair approach to shifting a greater proportion of the tax burden to very wealthy families. Who could object to a tax on large estates? But when a clever politician renamed it the death tax, public opinion shifted dramatically. Who could support a tax on dying?

Likewise, the power of a name is widely exploited by the food industry to promote the consumption of extraordinarily unhealthy products. How many people would want to eat something that contains, among other things, fruit juice, maltodextrin, sugar, corn syrup, modified cornstarch, dextrose, malic acid, mineral oil, acetylated mono- and diglycerides, artificial flavor, artificial color (red 40, yellow 5 and 6, blue 1), sucralose, carnauba wax, beeswax, and sulfiting agents? But call it Sunkist Mixed Fruit Snacks, and it becomes a bestseller among families who subliminally think that anything with the word "fruit" in its name can't be all bad.

Tony's mom used the power of a name to defuse their nightly battles over dessert. The idea came to her at a time when Tony, age thirteen, had made several healthy changes in his diet but continued to expect ("demand," according to his mother) a sugary treat after dinner. At first Tony's mother tried to break the dessert habit by waiting an hour after dinner to see if he would be willing to have something else instead. When that didn't work, she tried to redefine "dessert." "How about an apple?" she'd ask. "How about ice cream?" he'd answer.

It occurred to her one day that Tony had a very strong and specific association with the word "dessert." Drawing on his success in replacing unhealthy snack foods with healthy alternatives, she began asking Tony what he'd like for his evening "snack." She discussed the change with him, pointing out that his new snacks were healthier than his old desserts. Tony agreed to give it a try. "He immediately began thinking of other things to eat," his mom said. "If you can get away from the connotation, you can change the thought process." These days, Tony and his mom enjoy seasonal fruit, yogurt, or peanut butter on whole wheat bread after dinner and save the ice cream for special occasions.

Action Plan:
Call it like it is. Together with your child, make up names reflecting the actual ingredients of unhealthy products that have crept into your

diet. How about Frankenfruit for the item discussed earlier? Or, for the intrepid, how about renaming chicken nuggets "scraps-o'-chicken, pressed into natural-appearing shapes by machines, sweetened with high-fructose corn syrup, fried in hydrogenated fat, made to taste like real chicken with chemicals from a factory, colored with more chemicals from a factory, kept from rotting by even more chemicals from a factory, and frozen for months to years"? Admittedly, this one's a bit dramatic and doesn't exactly roll off the tongue. Make up your own names: it's fun and can be surprisingly effective.

Don't Stress About It

We used to think that mental stress — depression, anxiety, and low self-esteem — had nothing to do with our physical health. But now we know that our feelings can have a powerful effect on our bodies and our weight.

Mental stress can set in motion a sequence of biological changes that cause us to store more fat. Certain hormones are part of our evolutionary response to stress. These stress hormones prepare us to take physical action ("fight or flight") by raising our blood pressure and heart rate and flooding our blood with glucose so that we have a ready supply of energy. The response served our hunter-gatherer ancestors well, say, if they confronted a wild boar in the forest. In our increasingly hectic society, mental stress has become ever more common, but our ability to release it, especially by physical activity, is ever more limited. As a result, stress hormone levels remain persistently elevated. Over time, this can cause a number of chronic disorders, including increased body fat in the most dangerous location, the abdominal area.

Researchers in Finland studied 20 pairs of identical twins in which one twin was obese and the other of normal weight. The average difference in body weight within the pairs was about forty pounds. The obese twins with the most abdominal fat showed more evidence of stress — including high alcohol consumption, poor sleep quality, low energy, and psychological problems — than their lean twins. In addition, the obese twins with the most abdominal fat produced more of the stress hormones cortisol and norepinephrine. Interestingly, obese twins with fat located elsewhere in the body (not in the abdominal area) did not show signs of stress or elevated hormones compared to their lean twins.

Action Plan:
We may not be able to eliminate stress from our lives, but we don't have to suffer from its chronic effects.

- Before beginning each meal, take a moment with your child to breathe and relax.
- Encourage your child to take a break from homework or other activities when feeling stressed.
- Make regular physical activity a part of your family's lifestyle.
- If your child is showing persistent signs of major stress (wide emotional swings, declining school performance, social withdrawal, and lack of enthusiasm for life), consider seeking support from a specialist in child behavior.

I Have a Dream

Having a dream, goal, or vision for the future can powerfully shape our daily behaviors. For children struggling with their weight, this might mean visualizing themselves at a healthy weight and imagining all the possibilities that could follow.

Ashley's dream of being a soccer star like Mia Hamm helps her resist junk food. Ashley, who's ten years old, says that before coming to OWL, she always felt hungry. She ate with abandon, allowing herself unlimited bowls of sugary cereal in the morning, frequent treats, and second and third servings at dinner. Working with an OWL social worker, Ashley learned how bringing her dream into the present could help her make better food choices. She now keeps a favorite photo of herself wearing her soccer uniform taped to her bathroom mirror, which reminds her why it is important to eat right. And if she is tempted by an unhealthy snack or finds herself going for seconds, Ashley stops and checks in with herself. "Before, I thought I was hungry," she said. "Now, I know I'm not so hungry. I ask myself, 'What do you want: a yummy treat or to be like Mia Hamm?' I think it would give me more pleasure to be like Mia Hamm."

Action Plan:
You know how kids naturally plaster their bedroom walls with posters? Suggest that your child make a "dream collage" consisting of pictures, photos, drawings, words, souvenirs, an image of a role model or some special place — anything inspiring and meaningful that moves her closer to her goal.

BEN'S STORY

❖ When Ben first came to the OWL clinic, his weight was edging toward 270 pounds. He was known to his peers as "Big Ben," and despite having many friends, he sometimes felt lonely. He ate out of boredom or when school stress got to him. But Ben wanted to lose weight because he was uncomfortable with his looks and wanted to improve his sports performance.

Fortunately, Ben had three key factors on his side: a keen interest in athletics, a supportive family, and a generally happy outlook on life. All in all, he seemed like the type of person who would do well with some basic dietary changes. At the time, Ben was skipping breakfast each morning, eating leftovers off his friends' plates at lunch, and indulging in a chocolate chip muffin washed down with Gatorade most afternoons. For dinner he ate large portions of refined starchy foods and very few fruits and vegetables.

We gave Ben and his family a crash course in healthy eating and explained how small changes could lead to big results, especially since he was already so physically active. Ben left that first visit to OWL armed with recipes, shopping lists, and healthy eating tips and full of enthusiasm to renounce his unhealthy diet.

The first month, Ben followed the plan and lost three pounds. Subsequently, however, the weight piled on: five pounds at his two-month visit and another five pounds by his six-month checkup. Ben admitted that his afternoon muffin habit had returned and that he was now drinking up to seven glasses of Gatorade each day — the equivalent of twenty teaspoons of sugar. "I've gone back to my old ways," he said sadly.

As Ben continued to struggle with his weight, his parents, described by one staff member as "willing to jump over the moon for Ben," wondered what they were doing wrong. We assured them they weren't doing anything wrong.

Then, in Ben's junior year, the soccer team won the state championship. The year before, he had been cut from the team because he couldn't finish a two-mile qualifying run in time. "Those were the kids I used to play with," Ben observed. "I could have been a champ, but I'm not." Ben realized that his weight had kept him from participating in something he loved and vowed not to let that happen again.

At his eight-month visit, Ben decided to get back on track with his diet. Together with our staff, he devised a plan for proceeding "piece by piece," as he explained it. He gave up the chocolate chip muffins for good. Then he eliminated the Gatorade. He began to eat healthier foods that filled him up: a sandwich on whole grain bread for lunch, two apples for a snack, and a plateful of vegetables with lean protein for dinner. Finally, he limited treats to a weekly ice cream outing with his family. Ben also agreed to see one of our psychologists, who showed him techniques for dealing with school stress.

Since then, Ben has made steady progress. At his ten-month visit, he had lost seven pounds. At twelve months, another seven pounds had come off. Today, one year after the soccer team's big win, Ben has lost a total of twenty pounds. He has more energy, improved stamina, and better self-esteem. As he looks toward college in the fall, he plans to play intramural sports and is devising ways to resist the temptations he knows will surround him.

Ben, it turns out, is a champ after all.

Living in the Moment

Suppose you're heading to a meeting with an important client. On the drive, you're stopped by a red light. Waiting for the light to change, you begin to worry about being late. You look at your watch and think you should have left home earlier. You realize that you've missed the last three lights and wonder if it's a bad sign for the day. You see an elderly man in the crosswalk; he seems to be taking forever to get across the street. You notice a sports car in the next lane and hope it doesn't try to cut in front of you when the light changes. You look back at your watch and can't believe how long the light is taking. Finally, the light turns green. You accelerate rapidly to make up for lost time but have to slow down because of traffic. You arrive at the meeting five minutes late, tense and distracted.

Now suppose you're back at the light. When you begin thinking about being late, you take a deep breath and let it out with an audible sigh. You notice a cool breeze coming in the window. You feel your body relaxing. The sight of an elderly man in the crosswalk brings a smile to your face: he's dressed just like your grandfather. Still smiling, you catch the eye of a driver in the next lane. He smiles back. The light changes, and you head on to the meeting. You arrive five minutes late, feeling calm and fresh.

The difference between these two scenarios is mindfulness. Being mindful is a means for bringing ourselves into the present, the only moment in which life can truly be lived. You are being mindful right now as you read the words on this page, letting go of other thoughts and bringing your attention here. Mindfulness helps us respond to the world intelligently rather than reacting unconsciously. In the process, we are freed from endless worries and distractions and can experience life in all its richness and beauty.

Many religions, including Buddhism, have cultivated practices for being mindful. But we needn't live on a mountaintop or meditate daily to enjoy mindfulness. And we don't have to wait for a moment of peace to be mindful; mindfulness brings moments of peace to our lives. Mindfulness is always available to us, with each breath.

What does mindfulness have to do with eating and weight management? Consider another study by Cornell's Brian Wansink and his colleagues. They served 54 young adult volunteers a soup lunch in either green or blue bowls, encouraging them to think that the purpose of the study was to examine the effects of color on taste and perception. Unbeknownst to the volunteers, half of them had bowls attached to an apparatus under the table that imperceptibly added more soup as they ate. Afterward, the researchers asked the volunteers to rate how satisfied they felt and how much soup they believed they had consumed. Those who had eaten from the self-refilling bowls consumed 73 percent more soup than those who had eaten from normal bowls. Of particular interest, they did not believe they had consumed more, nor did they report being more satisfied than those who had eaten from normal bowls. The findings held true for both thin and obese volunteers.

This study shows that the amount we eat has little to do with how much we enjoy our food. If we eat mindfully, a bowl of strawberries with 100 calories can be more pleasurable than a bag of chips with five times as many calories. (And who among us hasn't eaten a bag of chips without actually tasting a single one?) When it comes to dessert, most of our enjoyment comes from the first few bites, whereas most of the calories come after that. As Susan Albers, author of *Eating Mindfully,* explains, "Mindful eating is less about *what* you eat and more about *how* you eat. You can even eat chocolate in a mindful way."

Action Plan:

- Conduct a mindful eating meditation with chocolate. Purchase some really good-quality chocolate. Sit down with your child at a table or on the grass. Breathe and relax for a moment, then give him a small piece of chocolate and take a piece for yourself. Ask your child to describe its color, texture, and smell. Ask him to imagine how it will taste. Then ask him to eat the chocolate very slowly, and you do the same. Notice how it feels on the tongue

---

NOURISHING TRADITIONS

❖ In the 1970s, nutrition researchers were puzzled that women in Thailand had low rates of iron deficiency even though their diets tended to be low in this nutrient. So they studied a group of Thai women under two conditions: eating typical foods served as a traditional meal and eating the same foods all blended together and therefore much less appealing. It turns out that the women absorbed more iron from the traditional meal, even though both meals contained exactly the same amount of iron. The study suggests that when we get more enjoyment from the foods we eat, we also get more nourishment.

---

and how it begins to melt. Can you detect a hint of bitterness, or perhaps even saltiness, along with the sweetness? When you swallow, notice how the chocolate travels down your throat and into your stomach. Afterward, discuss your experiences. Now eat just one more piece of chocolate together, again slowly, and this time in silence.

• Show your child what happens before food arrives at the table. Take her shopping for fruits and vegetables or, better yet, to a farm to pick strawberries in season. Prepare a dish together using these items. When children become mindful of where food comes from, they often develop a deeper appreciation and enjoyment of it.

• Eat a meal while being mindful of the sensation of fullness. Before beginning a family meal, ask each person to say how full he or she feels, on a scale of 1 to 10 (1 being not full at all and 10 being uncomfortably full). Then proceed with the meal, eating slowly and paying attention to sensations in the body. Every five minutes, ask family members to pause and describe their feelings of fullness on the ten-point scale. Whenever someone reaches a 7, encourage him or her to stop eating and sip a cup of tea until the rest of the family is finished. Then have a very light dessert together, such as half a piece of fruit per person.

Everything in Its Time

For everything, there is a season . . .
A time to plant, and a time to reap . . .
A time to weep, and a time to laugh . . .
A time to mourn, and a time to dance . . .

— Ecclesiastes 3:1–4

Sometimes, despite our best efforts, nothing seems to work out. We plan to make big changes, summon our energies, and charge ahead, but soon we run out of steam. Determined to eat right, we prepare dinners at home three nights straight, only to pick up a bucket of fried chicken, fries, and a sugary drink after a frustrating day at work. Intent on becoming more fit, we purchase a family membership to the local YMCA but somehow never find the time to go. At these times, it may feel as if we're running a race underwater while everyone else is running on land, or as if we're stuck in neutral when we want to accelerate forward. After a while, we become discouraged and wonder what's wrong with us. Eventually, frustration can give way to hopelessness.

At these times, it is especially important to be patient and gentle with yourself. Lower short-term expectations while taking basic protective measures to prevent things from getting worse. For instance, until you are able to begin a fitness program at the gym, take a ten-minute walk every day. Then give yourself time for things to change. For Ben, whom we met earlier in this chapter, it took eight months for the change to happen. For Peter, it took much longer.

THERE'S NO GOING BACK

❖ Addicted smokers wonder how they could possibly get by without cigarettes. But once they've kicked the habit and discovered how much better they feel, there's often no going back. The same can be true for children accustomed to junk food and TV.

When sixteen-year-old Kayla first came to OWL, she was eating a standard adolescent diet that included lots of sugary soda and juice. But she was very motivated and enthusiastically embraced our eating plan. At her six-week follow-up visit, she had lost nine pounds. "I can't imagine ever going back to my old way of eating," she said. "Last night, we went out to dinner, and I had a sip of my sister's Coke. It was so sweet, and I thought, *I can't believe I ever liked the stuff.*"

Ten-year-old Rachel discovered the joys of a physically active lifestyle, including regular biking, swimming, playing basketball and soccer, and gardening. After six months in OWL, she said, "TV doesn't seem as interesting to me as it used to be because of all the new sports and outdoor activities I'm doing. TV now seems plain and boring."

Peter came to OWL at age seventeen, largely at his mother's urging after a recent visit to the pediatrician revealed high cholesterol, high triglycerides, and a BMI that was well into the obese category for an adult. Weight problems, heart disease, and diabetes run in his family, and Peter's father, a pharmacist, was quite heavy himself. Despite some reluctance, Peter felt that he could benefit from our program and agreed to give it a try.

Initially, Peter worked to improve the quality of his diet, in particular by limiting his consumption of pizza and Chinese food when he was out with his friends at night. He was rewarded for these efforts by losing several pounds. However, a couple of months later, Peter took a job delivering Domino's Pizza and found himself giving in to temptation at work. Throughout the next year, his weight either stayed the same or increased somewhat. Nevertheless, he continued to see an OWL dietitian and a psychologist, focusing on ways to increase his motivation.

When Peter came to see us eighteen months after starting OWL, he was very frustrated. "I can't put my finger on why exactly I'm having difficulty," he said. He cried during much of the visit, feeling unable "to sustain motivation or stick with the plan."

Shortly thereafter, something changed. Four months later, Peter had lost fourteen pounds, and three months after that, he'd lost another twelve. At his last visit, Peter had lost a total of sixty-five pounds, two thirds of the way to his optimal body weight. A repeat blood test showed that his cholesterol and triglycerides had fallen into the normal range.

As we reveled in his accomplishments, I asked Peter how he had been able to turn things around so dramatically. He said that nothing specific had happened. One day, he said, "I just realized that it was ultimately up to me to do something about my weight." And he "decided to take ownership" of the situation. So he became "teammates" with his dad and joined the gym. He cut way back on junk food and reduced his portion sizes. Although he still has a way to go, Peter now reports feeling much better overall and being motivated to continue his weight management efforts. He said he was grateful to have had the help of his parents and the OWL Program when the time was right.

PART III

Making Peace
in Our Families

6

THERE'S NO PLACE
LIKE HOME

Once upon a time, there was a town that cared deeply for each and every one of its children. There were safe parks for kids to play in and tree-lined paths for them to walk. At school, regular breaks gave students a chance to exercise their bodies and relax their minds. School lunch was prepared fresh each day from the bounty of nature and included locally grown produce whenever available. Most nights, children ate dinner at home with their parents and siblings, nourished by good food and time together. When a stranger came to town trying to sell candy to the kids, he was told in no uncertain terms by the town leaders that such behavior was not tolerated.

Perhaps someday we'll all live in a modern version of that town. (Chapter 8 tells the stories of five people who are trying to bring that about.) For now, however, the family remains the last bastion of protection for our children in a world seemingly designed to make them fat. In this chapter, we offer OWL-tested techniques that can help families live peacefully in the home and empower children to act wisely outside it.

Parenting Through the Ages

Generally speaking, it's easy for parents to discipline defiant children at age four, much harder at age fourteen, and practically impossible once they've grown up and left home. Ultimately, the best way to influence children over the long term is through the strength of the parent-child relationship. In this relationship, the child progressively learns values that guide behavior for a lifetime and that are in turn passed down to the next generation.

Building a strong parent-child relationship can be challenging for any family in America today and especially difficult when a child has a weight problem. To build this relationship, we must tailor parenting practices to the changing needs of children as they grow. What is appropriate at one age won't necessarily work at another. Like newly hatched ducklings that "imprint," or follow and imitate the first thing they see (usually the mother), young children are biologically primed to learn from their parents. In contrast, adolescents seem almost hardwired to do the opposite of what their parents say. Keep in mind that your teenager still needs you very much, although he also needs to establish a measure of independence and carve out an identity apart from the family.

When it comes to behaviors affecting body weight, some parents raise young children permissively, perhaps in reaction to excessive strictness they experienced in childhood. But if parents don't provide firm limits and guidelines, our commercial culture will happily fill the vacuum. The extremely unhealthful eating and activity habits taught by TV and other media become deeply ingrained over time, often contributing to a weight problem by adolescence. At this point, parents become alarmed and try to clamp down. But strict limit setting at this developmental stage usually makes matters worse, resulting in an escalating power struggle.

The key to successful parenting is to establish a parent-directed system that provides firm limits and guidance when the child is young.

Over time, these limits are gradually released as the child matures, giving rise to a child-directed system that encourages autonomy and responsibility. With proper parenting practices, we can avoid many of the problems that commonly occur in families with overweight children and possibly help prevent overweight from developing at all. When conflicts do occur, effective parenting practices help us avoid making matters worse and begin to turn things around. Before we consider these practices individually, let's have a look at the unique challenges at four key stages of child development.

Early Childhood (Ages Two to Five Years): Setting the Stage

Tanya was deeply concerned about her son, Carl. At the age of five, his weight had climbed off the growth chart. He was suffering from high cholesterol and showing early warning signs of type 2 diabetes. Tanya knew that his diet of fast food, sugary cereals, and up to six cups of juice a day was fueling the weight gain. But whenever she served healthier foods for dinner, Carl would scream, thrash around on the floor, and refuse to take a bite. As a single mother with a full-time job, Tanya felt too tired at the end of the day to deal with her son's tantrums and overwhelmed by the nightly food fights. More often than not, she gave in to his demands.

Children are born with a preference for the primary flavors of breast milk — sweet, fatty, and salty — and are reluctant to try new foods. This natural reluctance, called neophobia ("fear of things new"), keeps young children from eating anything that could be poisonous. But if young children never developed a liking for new foods, they would starve after weaning. So nature has also primed them to learn eating habits by watching others around them, especially their parents.

Leann Birch at Pennsylvania State University and colleagues studied the responses of two- to five-year-olds to new foods under three conditions: in one condition, an adult was present but not eating; in another condition, an adult ate a food that was a different color than the child's food; and in a third condition, an adult ate a food that was the same color as the child's food. As expected, the children were more likely to eat the new food when an adult ate a food of the same color.

Other research by Birch has shown that when a child learns to eat one new food (spinach, for example), she will more likely eat other similar new foods (various green leafy vegetables).

Taste preferences are more easily influenced in early childhood than during any other stage of life. In the normal course of events, preferences broaden over time to include a wide range of flavors and textures, including fruits and vegetables. Until very recently, young children found out about foods primarily from adults who had their best interests at heart. Problems occur when parents do not regularly model healthful eating habits and instead children learn what to eat from those whose motivation is profit — specifically, the makers of fast food, soft drinks, and other junk food. These products, designed to appeal to children's desire for sugar, fat, and salt, arrest taste preferences in an infantilized state, creating the perverse situation in which healthy foods are perceived as inedible. This sets the stage for great conflict: when a parent pressures a child to eat fruits and vegetables, he resists, demanding the junk food he's been "programmed" to want. This often means a tantrum. The unhealthful habits learned early in childhood from TV commercials and negative influences outside the home can persist for a lifetime, with potentially devastating consequences. The food industry, of course, knows this. That's why children's TV shows have become little more than a series of food commercials. So is it really any wonder that a child who regularly hears "Silly rabbit! Trix are for kids!" will become an adult who thinks that salad is just "rabbit food"?

Consider this: no species of mammal in nature allows its young to eat whatever they want. What would happen if a bear mother didn't teach its cub what and how to eat? The cub wouldn't survive the winter. Our modern nutritional environment can be as dangerous to children as an arctic winter is to the bear cub.

Fortunately, problems in early childhood can be effectively addressed by parenting practices discussed later in this chapter, including protecting the shared family environment, modeling, and saying no with love.

Childhood (Ages Six to Eight Years): Emerging from Home

Zach returned home from school with a smudge of chocolate on his cheek. "How was school today?" his mother asked. "Great!" he answered. "Anna is moving to China, and I got two doughnuts at her going-away party. It was also Michael's birthday, so we had cupcakes and juice. Then my teacher gave me a piece of chocolate because I solved a really hard math problem." Zach's mother was surprised. She worked hard to make their home a safe food haven, and although she knew that Zach would get an occasional treat at school, she couldn't believe that he was allowed to eat so much junk food in one day. She felt her control over her son's food and health slipping away.

Children at this age are increasingly involved with school and other activities outside the home, fostering social development but also making them susceptible to influences beyond the family. When it comes to nutrition, parents have less control than before, as children become exposed to new (often unhealthy) foods and eating behaviors by peers and unrelated adults. At the same time, children are developing more sophisticated reasoning skills. At this age, children often ask "why?" You may have to explain your decisions regarding food in greater detail. But children's developing cognitive abilities mean that they are capable of understanding basic concepts about nutrition and health. You might describe to your child the effects of too much sugar on mood and energy level, for instance, then ask her to notice and report back how she feels after a healthy snack and after a sugary snack. Many children are able to control how much junk food they eat if they understand why they should.

When it comes to body weight, family influence remains critical at this stage of development, as demonstrated in a study by Moria Golan and colleagues from Israel. The researchers randomly assigned 60 overweight children to two groups: one in which treatment was focused on them and the other in which treatment was focused on parents as the "exclusive agent of change." After one year, children in the parent-focused group lost almost twice as much weight as children in the child-focused group, even though they received no direct instruction from the researchers.

In addition to protecting the shared family environment and modeling, you can use a variety of parenting practices at this age to encourage the development of healthful behaviors, including positive reinforcement, anticipating obstacles, and empowerment.

The Tweens (Ages Nine to Twelve Years): A Time of Transition

Jill came to OWL at the age of twelve with an open mind and a strong desire to lose weight. She was teased about her appearance at school and couldn't fit into the styles of clothes that other girls wore. She decided it was time to shed some weight, and her mother, who was concerned about Jill's health and had suggested weight loss programs in the past, was thrilled. At first the program brought Jill and her mother closer. They shopped together for healthy foods and ate more dinners at home instead of in restaurants. They even walked around the high school track together several afternoons each week. Jill's BMI began to fall. But on one visit to OWL, Jill had reversed course. She'd stopped going food shopping and walking with her mother so that she could spend more time with her friends. Jill's mother felt frustrated by what she saw as Jill's lack of commitment to her health and the growing distance between them. She questioned Jill about what she ate at her friends' homes. This caused tension between Jill and her mother, who was surprised and hurt when her daughter began "pulling away."

Tweens can seem like young children one day, clinging tightly to their parents, and teenagers the next, snubbing family in favor of friends. Kids at this age seek a deeper understanding of themselves and their place in the world. Their bodies start to change, and their hormones begin to surge. Although this is a natural part of growing up, it can be awkward, uncomfortable, and embarrassing for many kids. They may feel out of control and unsure how to act. Michael, the nineteen-year-old we met in chapter 2, recalled the tween years as if they were a fun house mirror, distorting reality beyond recognition. "You're looking at yourself a lot differently, you're looking at a lot of other people differently, and you wonder if they're looking at you the same way," Michael said. Whereas your son may have turned to you for guidance just a few months ago, he now looks to his friends for support. His social network expands, and he becomes more susceptible to peer pressure and media influences and less influenced by you.

But it would be a mistake to underestimate the power of parents at this stage. Leonard Epstein at the University of Buffalo and colleagues looked at 142 families with eight- to twelve-year-old children who were participating in weight loss programs. The researchers found that the parents' weight loss was strongly linked to their children's weight loss. After two years, the children who did the best had parents who also did the best. The researchers attributed this finding in part to the effect of modeling: that is, when parents engage in healthful behaviors, they benefit and the child benefits, too. Another study by Epstein's group showed that obese children of this age who found their fathers to be more emotionally accepting (one of three parenting factors examined) lost more than twice as much weight after one year as those who found their fathers to be less accepting.

Tweens' increasing reasoning skills make them less likely to take what you say on face value and more likely to expect elaborate and compelling explanations for rules, as discussed in the *Handbook of Parenting,* edited by Marc Bornstein. The motto "Do what I say, not what I do" probably doesn't work well at any age, and especially not for tweens. Communicate your expectations clearly and monitor your child, but not too closely. Gradually relax limits and give your child more responsibility as appropriate. This will help her develop self-management skills that will prove valuable in many areas of life. Use the full range of parenting practices discussed in this chapter.

Adolescence (Ages Thirteen to Twenty-one Years): Initiating Independence

Sixteen-year-old Stacey burst into tears when she described a recent dinner at a restaurant with her parents. When she contemplated aloud ordering a pasta dish, her mom asked, "Honey, do you really want that?" And when she reached for a piece of bread, her dad flashed her mother a look that broadcast his disapproval louder than any words could. As an only child, Stacey was used to being the center of her parents' universe. Lately, how-

TACKLING THE TEASING

❖ Most overweight kids get teased about their appearance at some point. At the OWL clinic, these kids sometimes report that teasing doesn't bother them because they know the other kids are "just kidding around" or that the kids doing the teasing are "just dumb." The truth is, teasing hurts. If your child is being teased, you can help her by showing your love and teaching her constructive ways to respond.

School-Age Children
- When your child tells you that she is being teased, avoid strong displays of emotion, as this may cause her to overreact to the teaser. Instead, show empathy and acknowledge her feelings without judgment. You might say something like "That must have felt awful."
- Listen respectfully before responding, letting her know you want to understand what happened before you begin problem solving.
- Even young children can learn strategies for coping with teasing, such as self-talk (think about their positive qualities), ignoring the teaser (pretend the teaser is invisible; don't look at him or respond), and visualization (imagine being protected by a shield that deflects words harmlessly).

Tweens and Adolescents
- Tell your child that people who tease others often feel scared, unhappy, or bad about themselves.
- Teach your child how to stay calm in the midst of teasing. People who tease others are hoping to get a reaction. Role-play different scenarios with him.
- Help your child be better prepared in the future by writing down hurtful things that kids say and then coming up with ways to respond.
- Kids who can laugh at themselves often have an easier time with teasing. If your child has a sense of humor, suggest that he make a joke of it.

ever, their attention had grown "suffocating" as they monitored every bite she ate and recorded her weekly exercise sessions on a calendar, against Stacey's wishes. She knew her parents loved her and were concerned for her health, but their concern was beginning to backfire, as Stacey was gaining more weight at each subsequent OWL visit. "I feel like I'm under a microscope," she said. "Every time my dad gives me that look or my mom makes a comment about what I'm eating, it makes me want to eat more."

Adolescence is a time of dramatic physical, emotional, and intellectual development. At this age, social status changes, as the child transitions into an adult. The profound nature of this transition is marked by rites of passage in many religions and cultures — bar or bat mitzvah in Judaism, *quinceañera* in some Spanish-speaking cultures, vision quest in some Native American cultures, and walkabout for Australian Aborigines.

Because of these rapid changes, parenting an adolescent can be especially challenging and difficult. Most parents cite adolescence as the stage of their children's lives that concerns them the most. And it's no wonder. Your once-content child now challenges your every decision. He may begin to question rules and reject decisions viewed as arbitrary. As the *Handbook of Parenting* puts it, this is a normal way for teens to flex newly developed "cognitive muscles." Teenagers distance themselves from the family as they invest more emotional energy in their peers. This, too, is a normal process.

Conflict with parents can reflect teenagers' growing independence and self-assertion, but it also may stem from basic differences in perception. Mary Story at the University of Minnesota and colleagues surveyed 282 adolescent-adult pairs living in the same household regarding the family mealtime environment and the adolescents' mealtime behavior. They found that the pairs agreed on next to nothing. For example, the adults reported more frequent arguments and more TV viewing during dinner than the adolescents reported; the adolescents perceived that they helped make dinner more frequently than the adults perceived that they did. When it comes to behaviors affecting body weight, parents and teens may be living in entirely different worlds.

Parents often attempt to control their teenagers' behavior by tightening the reins, as Stacey's parents did by monitoring her every bite. But when it comes to weight management in adolescence, close supervision rarely succeeds over the long term and can prove counterproductive. In a striking illustration of this problem, the Minnesota research group found that boys who were encouraged by their mothers to diet were more likely to engage in health-compromising eating practices, including binge eating, fasting, and skipping meals.

Ultimately, the challenge for parents of adolescents is not to take anything too personally. Adolescence is a stage, not a rejection. Although your teenager may appear to want nothing to do with the family, he still needs to feel connected and loved. It's still appropriate to set rules at home. At the same time, it's important to recognize that parents have considerably less control outside the home and that attempts to clamp down may backfire. Indeed, the ability to make independent decisions will be necessary for the rest of your child's life — encourage this behavior while maintaining boundaries that teach about safety. Effective parenting at this age involves acceptance, structure, and support. Pick your battles carefully and be sure to focus critical feedback on the behavior, not the child. If you've been acting like a member of the food police, now's the time to turn in your badge.

"PARENTING THROUGH THE AGES" means working with, rather than against, your child's basic biological makeup. Ultimately, there is no perfect way to be a parent. You know your child best, and your approach will depend on a number of circumstances unique to your family. However, children raised by parents who respect their feelings and opinions but also set clear boundaries, called the *authoritative parenting style,* tend to be more responsible, independent, and adaptive than children raised with other parenting styles, including permissive (indulgent without discipline), neglectful (emotionally uninvolved and without boundaries), and authoritarian (strict without sensitivity to child's feelings). And according to recent data from one of the most comprehensive child development studies in the United States to date, children with authoritative mothers had just a 4 percent chance of being overweight in the first grade, compared to 10 percent for children of permissive mothers, 10 percent for children of neglectful mothers, and 17 percent for children of authoritarian mothers. Authoritative parenting provides the flexibility to adapt parenting practices to the changing needs of a child over time.

Whatever your current parenting style or history of conflict with your child, it is never too late to develop age-appropriate parenting skills to help you proceed more peacefully into the future. Let's consider some specific parenting practices that will help you do just that.

The Two Pillars of Parenting

What if you could permanently influence your children's behavior without their even knowing it? You can, and here are two ways to do it.

Protecting the Shared Family Environment

This is the most basic parenting practice — exquisitely simple yet exceeding powerful. It is considered in various ways throughout this book. Protecting the shared family environment means creating a home that supports the physical and emotional well-being of your child and other family members. With regard to weight issues, it means making healthful eating and physical activities natural and easy, and making unhealthful habits much less so. Week 1 of the 9-Week Program (see chapter 7) offers many ways to do this, such as eliminating junk food from the home, removing TV from the bedroom, and creating an active play center in one corner of the family room.

The great power of protecting the shared family environment is that everyone benefits: an overweight child is supported to lose weight without being stigmatized, a lean sibling acquires health habits that prevent a future weight problem, and a parent's high blood pressure and other heart disease risk factors improve. Creating a home free of temptations, be they candies in the kitchen or TV in the bedroom, removes one of the main causes of conflict between parents and children — as long as everyone follows the rules. If Dad brings home doughnuts, the kids will wonder why they can't have one, too. When parents apply one standard fairly to all, their credibility increases, and this parenting practice becomes most effective.

Modeling

This is the primary way that children have learned how to behave since the dawn of our species. Children are born primed and ready to follow the examples set by others, especially parents. This process occurs automatically whenever our children are around us. We model a healthful lifestyle simply by eating well and being physically active in their presence. But children don't distinguish between the things we want to teach them and the things we don't. They also learn to eat junk food and watch too much TV if we model those behaviors. Remember this simple principle: if you do it, they'll do it, too.

Children also learn by watching other important people in their lives, not just parents. If we model healthy habits to older children in the family, they will in turn model those habits to younger children, producing a trickle-down effect. Even the babysitter can act as a model: just as we'd ask her not to use improper language in front of our kids, we can reasonably request that she not eat junk food in front of them. Although parental modeling can still affect adolescents, peer influences tend to predominate.

As discussed earlier, when parents in family-based weight programs lose weight, their children do, too. This relationship is probably due to modeling. So let your love for your child motivate you: when you model healthful behaviors, everyone in the family benefits.

Strategies to Change Your Child's Behavior

If parents follow the previous two practices early and well, children should, in theory, acquire appropriate values and healthful behaviors, and there would be relatively little need for methods to change behavior. In the real world, however, things are seldom so simple. There is a limit to just how protective we can and should be with our children. And sometimes we don't give much consideration to parenting practices until problems develop. So strategies are needed to keep children safe in the short term and to guide their behavior over time.

Behavior change strategies fall into two main categories, coercive and constructive. *Coercive strategies,* such as nagging and punishment, are often the ones parents turn to first because they tend to work quickly. But these methods have several important drawbacks: they teach children what *not* to do instead of what to do, they leave children feeling upset (no one learns well when upset), and they take a toll on the parent-child relationship.

Food restriction and pressuring — that is, rigidly denying children certain foods while forcing them to eat others — are coercive methods that can be especially counterproductive. Leann Birch and colleagues found that when preschool children were pressured to eat, they actually consumed less of the targeted foods than when they weren't pressured. Conversely, according to another study by Birch's group, five-year-old girls whose mothers restricted food tended to eat in the absence of hunger when they were seven and nine years old. In a third study by this group, eating in the absence of hunger was linked to increased risk for being overweight.

Constructive strategies tend to take longer to work than coercive strategies, but they're more powerful over the long term, and they support the parent-child relationship. Praise, rewards, contingency management, and other related methods help children learn appropriate behavior and develop into responsible adults. The goal isn't to eliminate coercive methods entirely, as they may be needed from time to time, but rather to shift to constructive methods as the primary approach.

Praise: Whether a verbal compliment, an approving glance, or an appreciative hug, praise can be a powerful form of positive reinforcement. Praise brings attention to what a child is doing right and encourages her to do more of it. And unlike coercive methods, praise supports self-esteem. When offering praise, keep three principles in mind. First, focus on the desirability of the behavior, not the value of the child. Say "It's great that you ate all your vegetables," not "You're a good girl for eating your vegetables." Some behaviors are better than others, but the child is always loved. Second, provide a simple, clear message. If you say "It's great that you ate your vegetables, but why can't you watch less TV?" all the child hears is the "but." Third, be consistent: something that is praiseworthy today should be praiseworthy next week. According to Len Epstein, praise may be one of the most underused of all parenting practices. "Considering how inexpensive praise is, I'm amazed how rarely parents use it," Epstein said. Look for ways to praise your child regularly.

Rewards: Another form of positive reinforcement is rewards. A reward provides an opportunity to celebrate accomplishments along the way to a long-term goal and to let your child know that you recognize his efforts. When selecting appropriate rewards, remember that you're not offering a bribe for good behavior. Avoid money or costly items. For young children, consider a sticker or star chart; for older children, an inexpensive gift or a special privilege. In addition, avoid anything food-related (consider raising this issue with your child's teacher). What message do we send when we reward a good performance on a test with a Tootsie Roll?

Contingency Management (First This, Then That): You may already be using this behavior change method without knowing it. Contingency management means making one thing dependent on another, which helps children learn responsible behavior: "First finish your homework, then go play with your friends." Contingency management lets children know what you expect of them, while giving them a sense of control.

When using contingency management, focus on establishing appropriate priorities, taking care not to use food as a reward. To illustrate this point, researchers from the University of Albany in New York gave young children a pair of snacks under different conditions. In one condition, the children were told that they must eat the first snack in order to have the second (as a reward). In another condition, the children were simply instructed to begin with the first snack and then have the second snack. Before the experiment, children rated both snacks as equally tasty. Afterward, those who were "rewarded" for eating the first snack lowered their ratings of the first snack's tastiness. In contrast, those in the other condition continued to rate the first snack as just as tasty. The take-home message is this: when children hear "You have to eat your vegetables before you can have dessert," they begin to devalue vegetables. Instead, say "First we eat our vegetables, then we have dessert." The distinction is subtle but important.

Setting Goals: Often the choices that we make (such as having an ice cream) are disproportionately influenced by a momentary desire (for a taste of something sweet) rather than by what's truly important (being healthy and feeling good). Setting goals helps bring our behavior in line with our values. Whether these goals are short term or longer term will depend on your child's age. Younger children need modest targets and frequent positive reinforcement, such as praise and a star in a chart for one day without junk food. A teenager might aim for thirty minutes of physical activity five days a week for a month. When helping your child set goals, focus on patterns, not pounds. Once the behaviors are in place, the weight will follow.

Self-Monitoring: This practice helps us become conscious of our behaviors, appreciating what we've done well and nonjudgmentally identifying areas that need more attention in the future. In study after study, individuals who self-monitor lose more weight than those who don't. At the OWL clinic, we encourage patients to track food- and activity-related goals on a calendar. For a goal of swimming three times a week, the child would place a check mark on each day that he swam and add up the total at the end of each week. When the child returns to OWL with the calendar, showing that he has accomplished this goal, he receives a small reward. Adolescents may prefer to monitor their progress by keeping a more elaborate food and activity journal. These methods are easy to do at home: all you need is paper, a pen, and some time. To encourage honesty and consistency, praise your child for self-monitoring, whether or not he achieves his goal. If he doesn't reach his goal, reassure him that there will be new opportunities for success tomorrow or next week.

Anticipating Obstacles: Our society places many obstacles along the road to achieving a healthy body weight. Specific obstacles will differ according to your child's circumstances, such as the quality of foods served at her school, the habits of her friends, and recreational opportunities in your local community. Birthday parties may be a problem for young children, whereas adolescents may have difficulty when their friends go out for fast food. Together with your child, anticipate likely obstacles and come up with ways to deal with them. Role-playing these situations can help your child implement the solutions when the time comes. Later in this chapter, Bill Dietz discusses how to anticipate obstacles when a teenager goes out with friends for fast food. In chapter 7, we discuss how to use this method when tempted to eat out of boredom and when going to a party.

Redirecting: Earlier in this chapter, we discussed the importance of protecting the shared family environment, a parenting practice that removes unhealthful influences from our children's midst. However, as children grow, they are increasingly exposed to environments beyond our control: a restaurant, the mall, even a movie theater. When we can't remove unhealthful temptations from our children's midst, we can aim to redirect their attention from the temptations and teach them to do the same for themselves when we're not around.

Studies by Walter Mischel and colleagues at Stanford University in the 1960s and 1970s dramatically illustrate the significance of redirection. The researchers gathered four- and five-year-olds and placed a marshmallow in front of each. The children were told that they could either eat the marshmallow immediately or wait a few minutes and receive a second marshmallow. When the researchers left the room, some of the children, unable to control themselves, broke down and ate the marshmallow within seconds. But other children managed to hold off by directing their attention away from the treat. Some sang or talked to themselves; others simply covered their eyes or rested their heads on their arms for up to fifteen minutes. Interestingly, Mischel interviewed some of the children from the original experiment fourteen years later. He found that those who were able to wait the longest before having the marshmallow were the most socially competent, emotionally stable, and academically accomplished. This study suggests that redirection helps children resist immediate gratification in order to achieve their goals and that this ability is important for long-term success in life.

Empowerment: This is the term we use for letting children take responsibility and play a role in decision making in an age-appropriate fashion. Examples of empowering activities include letting younger kids help with shopping or preparing vegetables, and letting older kids choose and prepare a side dish for dinner. In fact, a study by Dianne Neumark-Sztainer and colleagues of middle and high school students in Minnesota showed that those who helped prepare family meals often consumed higher-quality diets than those who did not. When children feel trusted, they usually rise to the occasion and act responsibly. And when they act responsibly, confidence improves — an important outcome for overweight children who may suffer from poor self-esteem.

FAMILY MATTERS

❖ Diane and her father, Gerry, signed on to participate in one of our research studies armed with a close relationship and a pact: there would be no secrets about what they ate and no lies about how they felt during the six-month study. This honesty policy included the inevitable "slips" that were bound to occur. Gerry knew from past experiences with dieting how easy it is to let a minor setback turn into a full-blown disaster. So he told Diane that although an occasional slip was OK, if it happened, she "must get back in the game."

The pair began the study with loads of enthusiasm. They cleared their house of junk food and started walking together. But within the first two weeks, Diane slipped. She was unable to resist the sweets and chips that her friends ate whenever they spent time together. She really liked these foods, and she also wanted to fit in and not call attention to the fact that she was trying to lose weight. She discussed this with her father, and they decided that Diane could allow herself to eat small portions of these foods when out with friends.

In the meantime, Gerry stayed the course at home, following a healthy diet and doing more physical activity than he had in the past. When Diane was home, she followed her father's lead. By the end of the six-month study, Diane had lost about twenty pounds, and Gerry had lost a few pounds, too. He believes that giving his daughter permission to "be human and make a mistake occasionally" allowed her to succeed.

Gerry may not have known it, but he was also using a variety of important parenting practices, including modeling healthy behaviors, empowering his adolescent daughter to make decisions about food, and developing strategies to deal with obstacles. In addition, he helped prevent her from succumbing to all-or-nothing thinking, a concept discussed in chapter 5. All of these practices supported their close relationship, the foundation of all good parenting. "Everything is aboveboard," Gerry said. "Frankly, I am certain that this is the key to her success."

Saying No with Love: Although saying no may seem like a negative approach, it is instead a constructive approach, as long as it's done with love. In some ways, this behavior change method, the last we consider here, forms the foundation for all the others. If we can't say no to some things (such as junk food), we can't say yes to others (such as good health). Saying no is a necessary way to teach children appropriate limits and boundaries for their immediate safety and their long-term well-being. When using this method, follow three guidelines. First, remember that you're saying no to a behavior, not punishing the child: be firm and gentle. Second, establish clear expectations and be consistent. For parents who are separated or divorced, maintaining consistency can be especially challenging. As best you can, negotiate a mutually acceptable approach, then present a united front in the interests of your child. Third, look for at least as many ways to say yes as to say no. If you say no more TV, ask your child to name three things he'd like to do as an alternative. Can you say yes to one of them?

How Were You Parented?

Sometimes the way we were parented affects how we parent our own children. Consider these two stories from parents in OWL.

When Susan was young, her mother was always on a diet, constantly obsessed with what she ate. Her mother brought only diet foods into the home and drank only black coffee with artificial sweetener. She seemed more concerned with her weight, Susan recalled, than with her family, and she was "emotionally unavailable" to her children. As a result, Susan grew up feeling deprived of both nurturing and nourishment. When her own five children were born, Susan had trouble setting any limits around food, which she connected in her mind to the withholding of love. Not surprisingly, the children developed atrocious eating habits. By the time her daughter Katie, age nine, became seriously overweight, Susan began to see that in trying not to be like her mother, she had gone too far in the other direction. A better

SCHWARTZ SUPPORT:
HOW TO TALK TO YOUR CHILD
ABOUT THE WEIGHT ISSUE

❖ Sometimes parents avoid discussing weight issues with their children out of concern for causing emotional upset or precipitating an eating disorder. However, in our weight-obsessed culture, overweight tweens and adolescents are well aware of their problem. And being overweight is one of the strongest risks for developing disordered eating habits. So beginning a frank, sensitive discussion about this issue can be a great relief for your child, and it can help you work with her to prevent an eating disorder from developing. Marlene Schwartz, a clinical psychologist at Yale University, offers some advice for having this discussion.

- Speak openly to your child rather than remaining silent and letting her imagine what you are thinking.
- Tell your child explicitly that you find her attractive and that she deserves to feel good about her body.
- Teach her that eating well and being active are part of taking care of her body, just like brushing her teeth and getting enough sleep.
- Keep your weight-related comments focused on your child's behaviors. Praise her for going for a walk or choosing fruit for a snack. If she loses weight and wants to tell you about it, say that you are happy her weight is reflecting her behavior changes, and remind her that the number on the scale isn't the only way to measure success.
- Help your child notice ways in which she feels better as a consequence of her behavior changes — for example, having more energy or being able to run around with friends without getting out of breath.
- If you're worried that your child has become obsessed with weighing herself or is engaging in dangerous behaviors to lose weight (fasting, using laxatives or diuretics, vomiting, exercising excessively), say something to her immediately. Tell her that the

goal isn't to become thin at any cost and that none of these strategies work in the long term.

- Treat laxative abuse or vomiting the same way you would treat drug or alcohol abuse. Be very clear that these are dangerous behaviors and that you are watching to make sure your child does not engage in them. If she continues to do so, consult a health professional who specializes in eating disorders.

understanding of her childhood experiences led Susan to reevaluate her own parenting practices and begin to introduce appropriate limits around food.

Joanie had the opposite experience as a child, remembering a childhood home stocked with unhealthy snack foods and sugary drinks. She was allowed to eat whatever and whenever she wanted, virtually without limit. By the time she reached adolescence, Joanie was quite heavy, and she continued to struggle with her weight for some time. Mindful of her strong family history of obesity, heart disease, and type 2 diabetes, Joanie, who had become a personal trainer, vowed to be more "structured and disciplined" with her own children. Even so, her son Max developed a weight problem. At the family's first visit to OWL when Max was nine years old, we observed Joanie lecturing him about food in ways beyond the comprehension of a child his age. At those moments, Max would stare off into space or roll his eyes. After two sessions with our behavioral therapist, Joanie recognized that she was being too controlling with Max, leading him to rebel by overeating when she wasn't around.

All of us carry experiences of our childhood with us. Consider how you were parented and how those experiences may be influencing your approach to your child's weight issues.

THE IMPORTANCE OF SELF-CARE

❖ With dozens of obligations pulling parents in so many different directions, taking time for lunch can seem like a luxury. If we don't take care of ourselves, however, we'll be less able to care for others, and we won't be modeling healthful behaviors for our children. So consider the advice airlines give passengers in the event of sudden cabin decompression: "Secure your oxygen mask first, then help those around you."

The Dinner Table

Now that you know what to expect across the key stages of child development and have thought about a variety of parenting practices, apply your skills at the dinner table. The family dinner offers a unique opportunity to do the following:

- Make healthy eating normal.
- Maintain control over meal quality at least once each day.
- Counteract the nutritional nonsense taught to children at almost every turn.
- Enjoy time together as a family.

To avoid unnecessary argument at the dinner table, we recommend creating a clear division of responsibility. As the parent, you have final authority over which foods to keep in the house and what's for dinner. Serve all members of the family appropriate-size portions based on their age and energy needs. Your child can decide whether to eat what you've served. If he doesn't eat it, don't jump up to make him something else. If he wants more than one serving, allow him to eat until he feels satisfied, encouraging vegetables and fruits first. Make

SOUL FOOD

❖ From the dawn of civilization, food, culture, and religion have been inextricably linked. *Haroset* at the Jewish Passover dinner means so much more than spiced, chopped apples. If you were born in Turkey, baba ghanoush probably reminds you of home, not just a way of serving roasted eggplant. Almost always, holidays and cultural celebrations involve foods specifically prepared for the occasion and eaten with appreciation. Unfortunately, these traditions have all too often been forgotten in our fast food/fake food culture, to the detriment of body and spirit. The Bible says that the body is a temple. For some people, this simple wisdom can inspire a profound transformation in diet. Why not make the family meal a sacred event? Prepare and serve foods that embody the love you have for your spouse and children. Make the dinner table a warm and welcoming environment. Turn off the TV. Leave unpleasant emotions and unresolved conflicts at the dining room door. Consider how the meal not only feeds the body but also nourishes our deeper selves. Eat consciously and savor every bite. In this way, fewer calories may be more filling — and fulfilling.

only enough starchy foods for one serving for each family member. Serve desserts in modest portions, with no second helpings.

Research has shown that children who have regular family dinners consume more fruits and vegetables, more fiber, fewer fried foods, less soda, and fewer trans fats than children who don't have regular family dinners. In addition, they are less likely to be overweight. In my opinion, having dinner with your child most nights is one of the two most powerful ways to prevent or treat a weight problem. The other is turning off the TV.

As we all know, children are born without an instruction manual, and many of us did not have ideal role models as parents. Remember that parenting is a learning process, both for you and your child. Be patient and give yourself time as you explore the techniques presented in this chapter. Then get ready for the 9-Week Program coming up next.

GOOD FOR YOUR WAIST — AND YOUR WALLET

❖ A nutritious diet saves money over the long term in fewer doctor bills, prescription costs, hospital charges, and missed days of work. A study by Len Epstein and colleagues suggests that eating right saves money in the short term as well. The researchers tracked the diets of families with overweight children participating in a one-year weight loss program. They found that as the intake of low-quality foods went down, so did daily food expenditures, by almost $2 a day per person. The cost of those deceptively cheap burgers, sodas, and processed snack foods adds up over time — to billions of dollars in profits for junk food manufacturers and higher family food bills for you.

DR. DIETZ'S PARENTING PRESCRIPTIONS

❖ When it comes to childhood obesity, no one deserves the title "Father of the Field" more than Bill Dietz, director of the Division of Nutrition and Physical Activity at the Centers for Disease Control and Prevention (CDC). Here he offers some advice for parents.

1. *Parents need to parent.* Food-related responsibilities in families should go like this: parents are in charge of what foods are offered at home, and children can choose to eat it or not. If a child rejects the food, it is not the parents' responsibility to offer something else, because this gives the child undue authority. Although some parents may worry that the child will be hungry later on, he will not starve.

Children need to learn that the consequence of not eating what is offered is hunger, and hunger is a powerful motivator.

2. *Your eyes may be larger than their stomachs.* Parents often overestimate how much food a child needs. They serve a large portion and expect the child to clean her plate. A better approach is to start with a small portion and let the child ask for more.

3. *Keep junk food outside the house.* Keeping junk food outside the house helps you avoid conflicts with your child around food. If the food is in the house and is denied, it becomes a forbidden fruit that is extremely difficult to resist.

4. *Don't mix mealtime with TV time.* Mealtime is family time, a chance to come together, share news, and interact. It's harder to have a meaningful conversation when the TV is buzzing in the background. Watching TV during meals also may lead to overeating, especially by people who are already overweight.

5. *Don't justify new rules regarding food.* When changing the household rules to support an overweight child, many parents feel the need to explain why to the whole family. This creates two problems. It stigmatizes the overweight child, and it creates a perception that because one child is overweight, everyone else has to suffer. Parents can simply say that the family is going to be eating healthier from now on and state the new rules.

6. *No means no.* Sometimes when a child asks for an ice cream, the parent initially says no. The child nags and nags, and eventually the parent gives in. This teaches children that they can get what they want by nagging. If you have trouble saying no, buffer yourself: "If you ask me again, you'll have to take a time-out." You can also set a limit on how many times a child is allowed to make a request.

7. *Stay involved as kids get older.* It becomes harder to direct your child toward healthy habits as she gets older, but it's not impossible. Many parents don't even try to influence their teenagers' food choices out of a mistaken belief that

they have no influence at all. Staying involved can make a difference. Talk to your child about which foods to choose at school, and become more involved in what her school serves.

8. *Change your approach with teens.* You may have to explain and negotiate a bit more with adolescents when setting rules around food. This is normal, but it doesn't mean that the rules have to change. For example, if you don't want your teen to have sugar-sweetened beverages, keep them out of the house. However, recognize that teens can do what they want with their own money.

9. *Strategize with teens.* Adolescents can be very sensitive about their efforts to manage their weight, especially when going out with friends. You can help your adolescent develop strategies to use when he is at the mall, for instance, and everyone orders a burger, fries, and a soda. Rehearse various scenarios, such as ordering the smallest serving size and having a no-calorie drink.

10. *Support activity.* Encourage your child to become more physically active by finding activities she enjoys. Some children thrive on the camaraderie of team sports, whereas others prefer more solitary activities such as yoga, dance, or karate. Some kids enjoy structured programs, and others do not. Whatever your child enjoys, provide her with opportunities to be active.

7

THE 9-WEEK PROGRAM

Welcome to the program! We've been waiting for you and are glad you're here. We've distilled all the key lessons from chapters 3 through 6 into a fun-filled, action-packed nine weeks (or ten weeks if you count preparation). Each week, we'll take you step by step through a different set of lessons, activities, experiences, challenges, and games. The program has been designed to be gradual yet progressive, leading to the possibility of profound transformation. As you get started, please keep a few guidelines in mind.

- Follow the program as a family, ideally including everyone who lives at home.
- Take the program at your own pace. It's completely fine to repeat a week, do weeks out of order, or take a week off in the middle.
- Feel free to modify any aspect of the program to suit your family's needs. Nothing is written in stone.
- Begin each new week on a Monday and end on the following Sunday, unless you have a reason to do it differently.

- Every Sunday, meet together as a family to review the previous week and make plans for the next week.
- Most important, have fun!

The program begins with a week of preparation. During this week, you and your family will take stock of your typical eating and activity habits in the Preparation Diary (page 302), without making any lifestyle changes. This information will be used as a reference point for the next nine weeks.

Weeks 1 through 9 contain the following elements.

Highlight: Each week, we'll focus on a central theme: the clean sweep, breakfast, lunch, dinner, snacks, hunger, dessert, eating out, and celebration.

Featured Food: As discussed in chapter 3, eating right helps you control hunger, lose weight, and achieve optimal health. In this section, we'll show you how to change your family's eating habits and apply the eight principles of low-glycemic eating (see page 69) one step at a time.

Featured Activity: The best results in any weight management program occur when mouth and muscles work together. In this section, we'll take weight loss into high gear following the six-point game plan (see page 92) for getting active without having to "exercise."

The Steps: Here we'll focus on achieving specific goals related to the week's highlight, featured food, and featured activity. Starting from their typical habits determined during preparation week, family members will gradually "Step Up" or "Step Down" certain behaviors until the week's goal has been reached.

Monitoring: Each family member records his or her progress with the steps in a copy of the Weekly Diary (see page 304). Monitoring is an important part of the program, as it brings consciousness to eating and activity behaviors. Studies have shown that self-monitoring is among the most important determinants of how well people do when trying to lose weight. Each week, only behaviors relating to that week's steps are recorded. We suggest that the family meet on the last day of each week (usually Sunday) to review their diaries, discuss their progress, resolve any difficulties, and plan for the week ahead.

Rewards: Weight loss is a long-term goal. To maintain motivation, it's important to recognize and celebrate accomplishments along the way. Help your children stay the course with Program Points that they earn by achieving their steps and monitoring goals. They'll have several opportunities to earn Program Points each week, so they can work toward a variety of small, medium, or large rewards. Here are a few simple guidelines.

- Create a list of rewards with your child, assigning point values to small, medium, and large reward categories. (Note that the maximum number of points that can be earned for the entire program is 45.) A sample list of rewards and points needed for each category is provided on page 152.
- Keep track of each child's Program Points in his or her Weekly Diary. Kids can cash in Program Points for rewards whenever they reach the 5-, 10-, or 20-point categories.
- Rewards are intended as a recognition of accomplishment, not as a bribe. Keep them modest, focused on promoting healthful behaviors, and nonmonetary.
- Remain positive. If your child fails to earn Program Points one week, avoid criticism. Instead, encourage her to do better the next week.

A SAMPLE REWARD SYSTEM

❖ There is a total of 45 possible Program Points for the entire 9-Week Program.

Small Rewards (5 Program Points)
- Trip to local pool
- Going to mall with friends
- One-on-one time with Mom or Dad
- Equipment for a new activity (jump rope, basketball, Frisbee)
- Child chooses one item on the dinner menu one night

Medium Rewards (10 Program Points)
- Having friends sleep over
- Movie night
- Laser tag
- New book or CD
- Manicure or pedicure
- Bowling or miniature golf outing
- Trip to science museum, aquarium, or zoo
- Child chooses entire dinner menu one night (Parents make it as healthy as possible.)

Large Rewards (20 Program Points)
- Concert
- Sporting event
- New outfit
- Getting ears pierced
- Day at amusement or water park
- Dance Dance Revolution or other active video game
- Child chooses restaurant for dinner (excluding fast food)

Support: In this section, we focus on additional ways that parents can support their children to achieve their nutrition and activity goals, according to the principles considered in chapters 5 and 6.

Tip: Each week, we'll provide information, recommend an activity, or offer a suggestion to help make things easy, interesting, and fun.

PREPARATION WEEK

You can't get where you're going unless you know where you are. This week, we take a close look at the dietary and activity habits of each family member, focusing on those areas covered during the next nine weeks in the steps.

- Choose a typical week to get the most accurate view of everyone's lifestyle habits. Postpone making any changes in lifestyle until after preparation week.
- Give each family member a copy of the Preparation Diary and Weekly Diary, and read the instructions (pages 302–305).
- Each night of the week, gather as a family to record each person's foods and activities that day.
- At the end of the week, determine each person's typical habits, as instructed in the Preparation Diary.
- You will use this information for the steps in the coming weeks. (You may be surprised by what you find out this week.)

WEEK 1

Highlight: The Clean Sweep

As we saw in chapter 1, changes in the environment since the 1960s, affecting what we eat and the physical activities we do, are responsible for more than two-thirds of childhood obesity. Unfortunately, we may not be able to bring back the more healthful social environment of the 1960s anytime soon, but we can create an island of protection for our kids at home. Make this a family affair.

The clean sweep can be one of the most powerful and motivating ways to launch a weight loss program. Choose a day when everyone in the family can work together and have fun as you turn your home into a nutritional safe zone.

- Right after breakfast, assemble the family in the kitchen and explain the plan for the day.
- Go through the cupboards, cabinets, refrigerator, pantry, and other food storage areas. Remove all sugary drinks, chips, cookies, candy, ice cream, refined crackers, and other fake food that doesn't support your family's health. Throw them away. Just for today, don't worry about being wasteful: the health costs of eating those factory products are far greater than their purchase price.
- Take the family to lunch at a restaurant that serves healthy food, go see a matinee together, or do both.
- After lunch, go shopping together for real food to replace the fake food you tossed. Stock your home with fresh and dried fruits, vegetables, nuts, nut butters, beans, whole grain bread and crackers, brown rice, lean protein, and healthy snacks. For inspiration, see the recipes in chapter 9 and the shopping list on page 307.

Filling your home with real food creates abundance rather than the sense of deprivation that so often accompanies typical "diets." Plus, you'll be protected from the complaint "There's nothing to eat!" The clean sweep doesn't mean you have to give up sweets. Without that half gallon of ice cream in the freezer, an occasional outing to the ice cream parlor becomes a special treat.

Featured Food: Vegetables and Fruits
Nonstarchy vegetables (both cooked and raw) and fruits are at the base of the Low-Glycemic Pyramid (see Figure 3.3, page 68). They are loaded with nutrients from nature, low in calories, and filling. Aim for 1 or 2 servings at every meal and snack.

- Raw vegetables — 1 cup
- Cooked vegetables — ½ cup
- Fresh fruit — 1 small to medium (apple, pear) or ½ cup (grapes, fruit salad)
- Dried fruit — ¼ cup

Featured Activity: Screen Time

Just as removing fake food from your home makes room for real food, cutting back on sedentary activities makes room for physical activities. And the granddaddy of all sedentary activities for kids today is screen time — including TV, video games, and computer. Aim for a maximum of two hours a day (not counting computer-related schoolwork or other work).

The Steps

- *Step Up:* Vegetables by 1 each day to a goal of 3 servings a day for little kids and 4 servings for big kids and adults. For example, a teenager eating 1 serving each day (as determined during preparation week) would step up to 2 servings on Monday, 3 servings on Tuesday, and 4 servings on Wednesday, then continue 4 servings a day for the rest of the week.
- *Step Up:* Fruit by 1 each day to a goal of 2 servings a day for little kids and 3 servings for big kids and adults. One 6-ounce cup of 100 percent juice can count as 1 serving of fruit each day. (Avoid drinking more than this amount.)
- *Step Down:* Screen time — TV, video games, and computer (not counting time spent on homework) by one hour a day to a goal of two hours or less daily.

Monitoring

Keep daily record of:

- Vegetable consumption
- Fruit consumption

IT'S EASIER THAN YOU THINK

❖ Sooner or later, there comes a moment that all doctors working with overweight kids dread. We pause, take a breath, and utter the "v" word: vegetables. Suddenly, the mother trembles, the father dives for cover, and the kid erupts with some version of "Eewwwwww! Yuck!"

Of course, there's nothing in a child's nature that makes him hate vegetables. If there were, humans would have died of malnutrition generations ago. In my experience, hating vegetables is essentially an American trait. I never saw anything close to it during my travels through Asia, Europe, and South America. The problem is, there's no way creamed spinach from a can will compete with French fries from McDonald's. Vegetables don't have to be a battle, but they do have to be tasty.

Eleven-year-old Sam and his mother, Tricia, were generally pleased with the progress they had made during their first few months in OWL. He had made substantial improvements in his diet and was becoming more physically active. However, he simply refused to eat vegetables.

Tricia, who held a demanding job in investment banking, recognized that she was no Julia Child. "I'm not a great cook, and my husband's much worse," she said. Nevertheless, each night she dutifully prepared a balanced dinner consisting of a protein, a low-glycemic starch . . . and canned vegetables. She was frustrated that Sam wouldn't even give the vegetables a try. Cautiously, I said that I probably wouldn't eat them either.

I told Tricia that I understood how little time she had to make dinner but that making vegetables tasty doesn't take much time. "Heat up a skillet, pour in a liberal amount of olive oil, and toss in some chopped garlic," I suggested. "In a minute, your kitchen will smell like an Italian restaurant. Wash a generous amount of almost any fresh, green leafy vegetable — spinach, broccoli, mustard greens, collard greens, whatever. Place in a skillet, add a dash of salt, and stir over medium heat. In less than five minutes, you'll have a delicious side dish that you'd probably pay $8.95 for at that Italian restaurant."

I offered several other easy cooking methods: "Wash and slice a pound of zucchini, place it in a baking dish coated with olive oil, cover with your favorite red pasta sauce, and bake at 400 degrees F for twenty to thirty minutes, until tender. Or steam just about any vegetable, sprinkle with grated cheese, and enjoy."

As Tricia listened to these possibilities, her face lit up. "I don't know why I thought it was so complicated," she said. "That sounds great!" I asked Sam if these recipes sounded better than the current canned offerings, and his expression let us know they did.

- Time spent in front of a screen: TV, video games, and computer (other than homework)

Rewards

- Maintaining accurate records of vegetables and fruits consumed and screen time — 1 Program Point
- Achieving vegetable goal — 1 Program Point
- Achieving fruit goal — 1 Program Point
- Achieving screen time goal — 1 Program Point
- BONUS for no more than ten hours of screen time all week — 1 Program Point

Support: Protecting the Shared Family Environment

The clean sweep is one of the best ways to make your home a place that supports health just by your being there. What other things can you do to make healthy choices convenient and easy, and unhealthy choices much less so? Here are a few examples.

- Remove TVs from all bedrooms.
- How many TVs do you need in the home? Can you get rid of any?

- Place a stationary bicycle or other exercise device near any remaining TVs.
- Create a play center in one corner of the family room with indoor toys and games that promote physical activity.
- Put jump ropes, balls, roller skates (with safety gear), and other outdoor toys in a conveniently located activity box.
- If you have a driveway or backyard, put up a basketball hoop.

Tip: Wash It and Watch It Disappear

When you get home from the grocery store, take fifteen minutes to prep the produce. Wash and cut up raw vegetables such as carrots, celery, and bell peppers. Wash cherry tomatoes, but leave them whole. Put everything in a large resealable plastic bag and place it prominently in the fridge next to a yummy dip. Place clean, dry lettuce in a storage bag for an easy-to-make salad. Cut up melons and strawberries, put them in a bowl, cover with plastic wrap, and place prominently in the fridge. Rinse apples, pears, and peaches and put them in a bowl on the counter. Rinse grapes, put them in a large resealable plastic bag, and place it in the freezer for bite-size frozen treats. Prepping produce will save you time during the workweek and help it compete with conveniently packaged fake food.

WEEK 2

Highlight: Breakfast

People who skip breakfast may go fifteen hours or more without eating, putting a major stress on the body. Later in the day, excessive hunger causes overeating that more than makes up for the calories not consumed at breakfast. Eating breakfast not only makes weight loss easier, but also improves school performance and mood throughout the morning. In addition, a balanced breakfast gets your child well on the way to achieving the day's nutritional goals, all before 8:00 A.M.

Don't have time for a vegetable omelet with fresh fruit? A slice of whole grain bread and peanut butter will do. See chapter 9 for quick, nutritious breakfasts every day of the week.

Featured Food: Whole Grain Bread and Cereals
Highly refined breakfast standards such as a bowl of Frosted Flakes, a bagel, or a doughnut start blood sugar on a roller coaster ride that can affect hunger and energy level throughout the day. Substitute whole grain for refined grain products as much as possible, especially at breakfast.

- Make sure the first ingredient on the label includes the word "whole." (The word "enriched" is usually applied to white flour, not whole grain products.)
- Try a variety of whole grains in addition to wheat, including brown rice, millet, barley, quinoa, and buckwheat.
- "Stone-ground" bread tends to be better than bread made from finely milled flour. Whole kernel or sprouted bread (found in health food stores; you can actually see the intact grains) is best. Look for bread that has at least 3 grams of fiber per serving.
- Look for breakfast cereals with at least 4 grams of fiber per serving.

Featured Activity: Walking
Here are some great things about walking.

- You can do it almost anywhere.
- You don't need any special training or equipment.
- You can take it at your own pace.
- You get to bring along family and friends.
- It's relaxing.
- It's free.
- Walking thirty minutes a day at a moderate pace would burn off

about 50,000 calories over one year, equating to about fifteen pounds of body weight.

The Steps

- *Step Up:* To eating breakfast every day this week. (Brunch is OK on the weekend.)
- *Step Down:* Refined grains (white bread, white rice, refined breakfast cereals) by 1 serving per day to a goal of 3 servings or less daily.
- *Step Up:* Walking by five minutes every day to a goal of thirty minutes daily.

Monitoring

Keep daily record of:

- Breakfast
- Refined grains
- Time walking

Rewards

- Maintaining accurate records of breakfasts eaten, refined and whole grains, and time walking — 1 Program Point
- Achieving breakfast goal — 1 Program Point
- Achieving refined grain goal — 1 Program Point
- Achieving walking goal — 1 Program Point
- BONUS for walking one hour or more on any day — 1 Program Point

Support: Modeling

Modeling is a powerful way that parents can teach their children healthful behaviors. And when parents model these behaviors, their health improves, too. So let's reverse the parental plea "Do as I say, not as I do." This week, focus on eating right, being physically active, and limiting TV viewing yourself. You may find that your child needs to be told what to do less often.

Tip: Sweet Dreams
Some people who skip breakfast have the habit of eating too much late in the evening. As a result, they awake in the morning feeling sick to their stomach and not wanting to eat breakfast: a vicious cycle. To break out of this cycle, begin by having something very light for breakfast, perhaps just a piece of fruit. Over the next week, aim to eat progressively less late in the evening and progressively more at breakfast until you've established a healthy eating pattern. Then notice how easy it is to shed those few extra pounds — and how much better you're sleeping, too!

WEEK 3

Highlight: Lunch
Meals served in the school cafeteria tend to drag the quality of kids' diets down even lower than it already is — a sad comment indeed. Take control of the midday menu by helping your child get into the habit of having a home-prepared meal most days of the week. See chapter 9 for convenient, cool lunches he will want to bring to school.

Featured Food: Beverages
Often kids have sugar-sweetened soft drinks because they're thirsty, not hungry. The problem is, when those drinks are used to satisfy thirst, they leave hundreds of high-glycemic calories behind. Although 100 percent fruit juice has a few more nutrients and sometimes more fiber than soft drinks, it contains just as many calories, and those calories add up fast. Very few kids would eat twenty apples a day, but how easy is it to have four or five cups of juice containing the calories

from those twenty apples? The best way to satisfy the body's need for energy is food; the best way to satisfy the body's need for fluid is beverages without calories: water, seltzer water, no-calorie flavored water, and tea.

Featured Activity: NEAT Things to Do

Non-exercise activity thermogenesis — which results from the simple physical activities in our daily lives — can make a huge difference when it comes to weight management over the long term (see chapter 4). Sneak in physical activity in any of the following ways, or come up with your own activities.

- Take the stairs instead of the escalator or elevator.
- Walk rather than drive whenever possible. If you drive, choose a parking spot at the far end of the lot.
- Hide the TV remote control so that family members have to get off the couch to change the channel.
- Encourage your child to take a five-minute "stand and stretch" break every thirty minutes when she's working on the computer or doing homework.

The Steps

- *Step Up:* To eating a home-prepared lunch four days this week.
- *Step Down:* Fruit juice by 1 cup each day to a goal of at most 1 cup daily.
- *Step Down:* Sugar-sweetened beverages by 1 cup each day to a goal of none.
- *Step Up:* Water and other no-calorie beverages by 1 cup each day to a minimum of 5 cups for little kids and 7 cups for big kids and adults.
- *Step Up:* NEAT activity, replacing passive activity seven times this week.

Monitoring

Keep daily record of:

- Homemade lunches that you ate this week
- Beverages consumed (juice, sugary drinks, and water/no-cal beverages)
- Times that a NEAT activity replaced a passive activity

Rewards

- Maintaining accurate records of lunches, beverages, and NEAT activities — 1 Program Point
- Achieving lunch goal — 1 Program Point
- Achieving fruit juice goal — 1 Program Point
- Achieving sugary drink goal — 1 Program Point
- Achieving no-calorie beverage goal — 1 Program Point
- Achieving NEAT activity goal — 1 Program Point

Support: One Step at a Time

After just three weeks on the program, your child may feel as if completing all nine weeks will take forever. Remind her that many important things take time, consider how far you've come already, and commit to taking the next step toward achieving a healthy body weight. This may be a good time to cash in your child's points for a small reward.

Tip: The Power of Ten

If you have only ten minutes to be physically active, go for it. Those ten minutes count toward your daily total. If you don't have time to walk for thirty minutes, break it up into three 10-minute blocks or two 15-minute blocks. This is like dropping nickels and dimes into a piggy bank: no matter how you count it, you still have thirty cents. In just ten minutes, you can go for a walk around the block, give your energy level a boost, and put a smile on your face.

WEIGHED DOWN BY SUGAR

❖ It's one thing for adults to tell children that soft drinks contain lots of sugar. It's another for them to see it for themselves. Most regular soft drinks contain 10 percent sugar. That means there's 2 ounces of it in a 20-ounce bottle of soda: about 15 teaspoons! With your child, take an empty 20-ounce bottle and add 15 teaspoons of sugar, 1 teaspoon at a time. Tell him this is exactly what he's putting into his body each and every time he has one of those drinks. Also tell him that those calories add up to two pounds of fat every month. You may see a change in your child's beverage habits very soon.

WEEK 4

Highlight: Dinner

Dinner is the time when parents can guarantee the nutritional quality of at least one meal and simultaneously model healthful eating. Not surprisingly, children who eat dinner with their families have a higher-quality diet and tend to be thinner than those who don't. Plus, dinner provides an important opportunity for the family to come together — an increasingly rare event in our busy lives. Turn off the TV and discuss the events of the day or other interesting, pleasant topics. See chapter 9 for some dinner recipes.

Featured Food: Vegetarian Sources of Protein

There are many ways to get protein besides meat, eggs, and dairy. Vegetarian protein is cholesterol-free, is low in saturated fats, and tends to cause less insulin secretion than animal protein, providing benefits to cardiovascular health. Having more vegetarian protein and less animal protein is good for your body and good for the planet, too. Give the following foods a try. For more information, consult a vegetarian cookbook.

- Beans — including black beans, red beans, pinto beans, navy beans, garbanzo beans, and black-eyed peas. Can be used in soups, salads, and side dishes or as a main course. Try dipping vegetables in hummus or other bean dips for snacks.
- Nuts — including peanuts (technically a legume), almonds, walnuts, pecans, cashews, and macadamias. Eat them plain, roasted, or as nut butters.
- Vegetarian cold cuts, burgers, and hot dogs. Typically made from soybean and/or wheat protein; available in most supermarkets, often in the refrigerator or freezer section. Use in a sandwich instead of conventional cold cuts.
- Tofu. A highly nutritious protein made from soybeans; versatile and takes on whatever flavor you wish.
- Tempeh. Made from fermented soybeans; commonly eaten in Japan. Has a stronger taste than tofu and goes well with teriyaki sauce.
- Seitan. Made from wheat protein; has a breadlike consistency. Popular with vegetarians.

Featured Activity: Active Play
Kids can burn off calories and have fun without ever considering it "exercise."

- For younger kids: Jump rope; play hopscotch, tag, or hide-and-seek.
- For older kids: Play catch, capture the flag, or paintball; shoot hoops.
- For all ages: Dance, including video-assisted games such as Dance Dance Revolution.

The Steps
- *Step Up:* Foods with vegetarian protein by 1 serving per day to a goal of 3 servings daily.
- *Step Down:* Red meat to a goal of none this week.
- *Step Up:* To active play four days this week for at least thirty minutes each day.

Monitoring
Keep daily record of:

- Vegetarian sources of protein
- Red meat consumption
- Active play

Rewards
- Maintaining accurate records of vegetarian protein, red meat, and active play — 1 Program Point
- Achieving vegetarian protein goal — 1 Program Point
- Achieving red meat goal — 1 Program Point
- Achieving active play goal — 1 Program Point
- BONUS for having one day completely vegetarian (dairy OK) — 1 Program Point

Support: Empowerment
Consider how to involve your child in decision making and how to reverse the normal power structure (as appropriate). Let your child:

- Participate in menu planning and food preparation. Generally speaking, if children cook it, they'll eat it.
- Take turns picking music for dinner.
- Choose a vegetable that you must buy, prepare, and eat yourself. (Kids have the option to eat this dish or not.)

DR. DAVID'S HEALTHY ASIAN DINNER
IN FIFTEEN MINUTES

❖ You probably won't be surprised that, as a doctor, I work late some nights. Last night, I arrived home at 8:10 P.M., and by 8:30 dinner was ready. Here's how I did it.

- Minute 1: Heat 1 cup water in a pot with a steamer basket. Wash and chop kale and carrots. Open a container of Caribbean-flavored tofu (available in most supermarkets; you can substitute other flavors) and cut into ½-inch-thick slices.
- Minute 5: Preheat a cast-iron skillet. Add 2 tablespoons olive oil and the tofu. Cook, turning every few minutes.
- Minute 7: Place the kale and carrots in the steamer.
- Minute 8: Place ½ cup leftover brown rice in the steamer. (Rice keeps well in the fridge for up to five days.)
- Minute 9: Place ¼ cup kimchee on a dinner plate. (Kimchee is Korean pickled vegetables. It is available at Asian markets and many health food stores. You can substitute regular salad.)
- Minute 10: Arrange a few dates and some roasted walnuts on a separate small plate. Set aside for dessert. Pour a glass of water.
- Minute 13: Place the steamed vegetables and rice on the dinner plate and drizzle with extra virgin olive oil and/or lemon juice.
- Minute 14: Place the tofu on the dinner plate.
- Minute 15: Enjoy!

Try creating your own fifteen-minute meal — and send me the recipe. I expect to have a few more late nights in the future.

Tip: And the Winner Is . . .

Let everyone in the family flavor his or her own version of tofu and then have a contest to see whose is best. Divide firm or extra-firm tofu into 4-ounce portions (one for each person), cut into bite-size pieces, and put in separate small, ovenproof dishes. Have each family member season his or her portion of tofu with soy sauce or salt and some combination of ginger, garlic, onion powder, chili powder, turmeric, cumin, peanut butter (diluted with water), or anything else that comes to mind. Add 2 tablespoons water and 1 tablespoon extra virgin olive oil or sesame oil. Mix and let marinate for 10 minutes. Bake at 350 degrees F for 30 minutes. Serve as the protein portion of a balanced meal and vote for the winner. Some dishes may be delicious; others may be disastrous. Give everyone credit for trying.

WEEK 5

Highlight: Snacks

Merriam-Webster's Collegiate Dictionary defines "snack" as "a light meal," and that's the best way to think of it. If you wouldn't eat cookies for dinner, don't have cookies for a snack. Save them for an occasional dessert after a balanced meal. Snacks provide a great way to nourish the body, boost metabolism, and keep hunger at bay between meals. Research suggests that people who have frequent, small meals and snacks weigh less than those who have less frequent, large meals. Encourage your child to have regular, healthy snacks — two or three each day for younger kids and one or two for older kids. See chapter 9 for suggestions.

Featured Food: Fats and Oils

Fats and oils used to be considered the least healthy nutrients in our diet. However, recent studies have clearly shown that the proportion of fats in a person's diet doesn't affect weight very much. In fact, certain types of fats actually lower our risks for diabetes and heart disease. And fats can make foods tasty: vegetables are more appealing when drizzled with olive oil, and salads are more satisfying with regular rather than fat-free dressing. When choosing among types of fats, read food labels and consider the following:

- Unsaturated fats — the healthiest type. Found in olive oil, canola oil, avocados, most nuts, and fish.

- Saturated fats — unhealthy when consumed in excess. Large amounts are present in red meat and dairy products.
- Trans fats (partially hydrogenated oils) — the worst kinds of fats, among the most toxic substances in the food supply. They are commonly present in many packaged foods and baked goods and in most deep-fried fast food. Avoid any products that contain these factory-produced substances.

Featured Activity: Sports

Sports are a great way for kids to get active without having to "exercise." Check out what's offered at your child's school, the local community or recreation center, or the YMCA. Consider:

- Team sports — basketball, baseball, football, soccer
- Martial arts — tai chi, karate, tae kwon do, judo
- Noncompetitive sports — dance, swimming, biking, yoga, skating
- Charity walkathons (Train for them with your child.)

The Steps

- *Step Up:* To having 1 to 3 healthy snacks every day this week.
- *Step Down:* Items with trans fats by 1 per day to a goal of none.
- *Step Up:* To doing an active sport for at least thirty minutes three days this week.

Monitoring

Keep daily record of:

- Healthy snacks
- Trans fats
- Active sports

Rewards

- Maintaining accurate records of healthy snacks, trans fats, and active sports — 1 Program Point

- Achieving healthy snack goal — 1 Program Point
- Achieving trans fat goal — 1 Program Point
- Achieving sports goal — 1 Program Point

Support: Reducing Stress

It's so easy to get caught up in the stresses of modern life. Stress can undermine any weight loss program, unless it is released. Together with your child, do one or more of the following this week.

- Vigorous outdoor activity
- Walk in nature
- Yoga class
- Twenty-minute meditation listening to relaxing music
- Puppet show, trip to the zoo, nonviolent movie, or other pleasant diversion

Tip: Sit Down and Relax

You've seen it before: your child hangs on the refrigerator door staring inside while he munches on a bag of potato chips and complains there's nothing to eat. As cold air floods out, he's not just wasting electricity; he's wasting an opportunity to make a healthful choice. Help your child decide what to eat for an afternoon snack by coming up with a list of options with him at the beginning of the week and then stocking your home with those foods. Encourage your child to put the snack on a plate and sit down to eat it. He will end up eating less and enjoying the food more.

Week 6

Highlight: Hunger

It is said that Native Americans have twenty different words for corn and native Alaskans have twenty different words for snow. Perhaps we need twenty different words for hunger — ranging from that desperate feeling when our blood sugar is too low to that pleasant feeling when it's just time to eat. Hunger is our body's way of communicating that the fuel is running low. Paying attention to hunger between meals lets us know when we need a snack, helping us avoid overeating later. Paying attention to hunger during meals lets us know when to stop eating.

Help your child make a diary to record how hungry she feels every hour through one entire day. Have her rank her hunger from 1 to 10, with 1 being not hungry at all and 10 being starving. Also note the time of every meal and snack. At the end of the day, explore with your child if she became too hungry before eating or if she ate when she wasn't feeling hungry at all.

Featured Food: The Balanced, Low-Glycemic Meal

A balanced, low-glycemic meal releases nutrients into the body slowly, fills us up with fewer calories, and keeps us full longer. If your child tends to become hungry one or two hours after eating, chances are he didn't have a balanced, low-glycemic meal. Combine lean protein, a healthful fat, and a low-glycemic carbohydrate for a meal or snack that satisfies longer.

Featured Activity: Active Travel

Find active ways to get where you're going instead of taking the car, bus, or subway.

- Walk an errand instead of driving it.
- Get off the bus or subway one or two stops early and walk the rest of the way.
- If it is safe, have your child pick one or two days each week to walk, bike, skate, or skateboard to school (wearing appropriate protective gear, including a helmet).

The Steps

- *Step Up:* To having a balanced meal at least twice a day every day this week.
- *Step Up:* To using an active travel method to get somewhere every day this week, weather permitting.

Monitoring

Keep daily record of:

- Which meals were balanced, low-glycemic meals
- Active travel methods

Rewards

- Maintaining accurate records of meals and active travel — 1 Program Point
- Achieving balanced meal goal — 1 Program Point
- Achieving active travel goal — 1 Program Point
- BONUS for having three balanced meals every day this week — 2 Program Points

Support: Anticipating Obstacles

An extremely common obstacle in weight management for children and adults alike is eating when not hungry, often out of boredom. If we're not hungry, that means our bodies don't need more food. This week, discuss with your child what to do when he feels like having something to eat between regularly scheduled meals and snacks. At those moments, we can ask ourselves the following question: Am I really hungry? If the answer is yes, have a healthy snack. If the answer is no, don't eat anything. Instead, do something interesting and fun — ideally outdoors and away from temptation.

Tip: Slow It Down

There is a point in every meal when we've eaten enough to be satisfied but are not uncomfortably full. The Japanese describe this point as being 70 percent full (or, for children, when there's still a little room left). Finding this point can take some attention, especially if we're accustomed to overeating. Many of us simply don't know how much food we actually need. One way to make this easier is to eat slowly, because it can take some time for the body to recognize and respond to the food we eat. By ending the meal then, we not only increase enjoyment (what's worse than that overstuffed feeling?) but also are well on our way to losing weight. Slow yourself down at meals by using these strategies.

- Put your fork or spoon down between bites and don't pick it back up until you have swallowed the food in your mouth.
- Eat with chopsticks.
- Chew your food well. Can you take thirty seconds for each bite? A minute?
- Make it a goal for meals to last at least thirty minutes when you have the time.
- Take less food than you think you need. If you're still hungry, you can always go back for more. Choose extra helpings of veggies and fruits first.
- Have an eating race. The last person to finish wins.

CHEW ON THIS

❖ Chewing may be the most underestimated of all physical activities. Researchers examined the effects of chewing in two groups of rats, one raised on standard chow and the other on soft chow that had the same nutrient composition but required less chewing. Both groups ate the same amount of food, but the rats eating the soft chow burned off fewer calories while eating than the rats eating the standard chow, and consequently, they gained more body fat. In humans, chewing gum burns about 12 calories an hour. At three hours per day, that could amount to four pounds of weight loss over a year.

WEEK 7

Highlight: Dessert

We're going on the record: we're in favor of dessert and recommend it every night! In fact, there are two important reasons to have a nightly dessert. First, dessert tastes good. Second, it brings dinner to a pleasant close, making for a transition away from the table and into the evening activity. Dessert can actually help you avoid overeating, as long as you keep in mind a few simple guidelines.

- Go for quality. A moderate-size piece of real chocolate can be more satisfying than a large piece of artificially flavored, fat-free "chocolate" cake with twice the calories.
- Eat consciously. Make half a piece go twice as far.
- Keep it light. Dessert isn't supposed to be a major source of calories, but rather a touch of something refreshing, rich, or sweet after a balanced meal.

Featured Food: Natural Sweets versus Sugary Sweets

Most nights, choose naturally sweet, healthy desserts rather than highly sugared desserts.

- Fresh fruit salad with a bit of honey
- Baked apple with cinnamon and nutmeg
- Small handful of roasted almonds and dates
- Real hot chocolate with a bit of real maple syrup
- Berries and yogurt with a bit of honey
- Cheese and real fruit preserves on whole grain crackers

Featured Activity: Active Chores

Here are some old-fashioned ways for kids to burn off calories. (Parents, you don't have to thank me for this!)

- Washing the dishes (by hand)
- Cleaning the house
- Gardening
- Mowing the lawn
- Sweeping the driveway or walkway
- Shoveling snow
- Helping buy groceries
- Doing an errand that involves walking

The Steps

- *Step Up:* To having a modest-size, healthy dessert after every dinner this week.
- *Step Down:* Sugary sweets and treats to no more than once this week.
- *Step Up:* To doing an active chore five days this week.

Monitoring

Keep daily record of:

- Healthy desserts
- Sugary sweets
- Active chores

Rewards

- Maintaining accurate records of healthy desserts, sugary sweets, and active chores — 1 Program Point
- Achieving healthy dessert goal — 1 Program Point
- Achieving sugary sweets goal — 1 Program Point
- Achieving active chore goal — 1 Program Point

Support: Avoiding All-or-Nothing Thinking

Remember, we don't have to be perfect in order to achieve our goals. If we overdo food or underdo activity, it doesn't mean we've blown it forever. Encourage your child to take setbacks in stride and get right back on track.

Tip: Just Give It a Try
Sometimes even thinking about doing something active can make you tired. On those days, commit to just ten minutes of physical activity. If you still feel sluggish after ten minutes, call it quits for the day, knowing you gave it a go. You'll likely find, however, that those ten minutes of activity provide just the energy boost you need to accomplish the rest of your goals for the day.

WEEK 8

Highlight: Eating Out
In case you were wondering, there are:

- 1,610 calories in a Double Quarter Pounder with cheese, large fries, and large Coke from McDonald's
- 1,950 calories in a large popcorn chicken, mashed potatoes, apple pie minis, and large Mountain Dew from KFC
- 2,510 calories in a Monster Thickburger, small fries, and vanilla shake from Hardee's

All of these foods come loaded with partially hydrogenated fats, highly processed grains or sugar, and not a fruit or vegetable to be found (unless you count that obligatory piece of tired iceberg lettuce on the burger). But eating out doesn't have to be a dietary disaster. You can enjoy healthy, balanced meals at restaurants and then enjoy how you feel afterward.

Featured Food: Restaurant Food and Take-Out
Here are a few simple restaurant rules.

- When it comes to the worst kinds of fast food (see above), just say no. If your child has it on rare occasions when she's out with friends, OK. But don't support this habit in any way. If she starts nagging for it on the way home from school, simply tell her, "This car does not make stops for fast food."
- Find quick service at takeout restaurants that offer healthier fare. It doesn't have to be a choice between an expensive French restaurant and McDonald's.
- When having dinner at a full-service restaurant, ask the waiter to bring the bread with the meal, rather than before. Those high-glycemic calories have their greatest impact on an empty stomach. Encourage everyone to have a salad and a cooked vegetable. Order one dessert for every two people.
- Make eating out a special occasion, not a regular event.

Featured Activity: TV Turnoff Week

As we discussed in chapter 4, TV "programs" children to gain weight in three ways. First, kids burn off fewer calories watching TV than doing virtually anything else. Second, mindless eating is all too common in front of the TV. Third, and perhaps most important, food commercials brainwash kids to consume fast food, sugary drinks, and other extraordinarily poor-quality products — undermining our efforts as parents to encourage healthy eating.

- Have a TV-free week. Turn the TV off for the entire week. (Yes, you can do it!)
- Rediscover how families spent time together before the 1960s:
  - Pack up dinner for a picnic in the park or at the beach.
  - Go for a walk or bike ride after dinner.
  - Play an outdoor game of Frisbee, badminton, or miniature golf.
  - Play a board game or perhaps a game of charades.
  - Listen to a radio show.
  - Read a book or go to the library together.

- Have family friends over for an evening of good conversation (parents) and active play (kids).

The Steps

- *Step Up:* To having a salad, cooked vegetable, or fruit at every snack or meal away from home this week.
- *Step Down:* To no TV all week.

Monitoring

Keep daily record of:

- Meals away from home
- TV time

Rewards

- Maintaining accurate records of meals away from home and TV time — 1 Program Point
- Achieving meals away from home goal — 2 Program Points
- Achieving TV goal — 3 Program Points
- BONUS for no fast food all week — 2 Program Points

Support: Saying No with Love

As a parent, it's OK to have rules and say no — it comes with the territory. The irony is that the better we get at saying no, the less we have to say it. For example, you can say no to your child once when she asks for ice cream in the market or night after night when she asks for it at home. Just keep a few simple guidelines in mind.

- Let no mean no. If a child learns that she can get what she wants by nagging, you're sunk.
- You don't have to justify yourself to your child. For example, you can simply say that house rules don't allow junk food inside.
- Make sure that your child understands that saying no isn't a form of punishment. Apply the rules fairly to all.

- Find creative ways to say yes at least as often as you say no. For example, is there a healthier alternative to the carton of ice cream that your child would like?

Tip: Don't Be Afraid to Ask
Many restaurants will happily accommodate special requests. Ask for:

- Olive oil instead of butter for bread
- A wedge of lemon to make the table water tastier (instead of ordering soda)
- An extra serving of salad or cooked vegetables instead of a refined starchy food
- The entrée to be broiled or sautéed instead of deep-fried
- Fresh fruit or berries for dessert (And these don't have to be shared!)
- Half of your entrée to be wrapped to go when you place your order

WEEK 9

Highlight: Celebration
Congratulations, you've finished the 9-Week Program!

- Celebrate all that you've done together as a family these past nine weeks, everything you've learned, and the many healthful changes you've made. Look back at each family member's Preparation Diary to see just how far you've come.
- Consider which lifestyle changes you'd like to make permanent and how you can do it.
- Connect with others outside the family to enlist their support. Broaden opportunities to improve nutrition and access to physical activities in your school, your community, and the environment at large.

Featured Food: Party Foods
Together with your child, use the parenting practice anticipating obstacles when it comes to parties.

- Plan for your child to have a balanced meal or snack before arriving at a party so that he doesn't arrive too hungry.
- Teach him to identify and choose natural foods such as vegetables, fruits, cheese, and nuts first.
- Tell him it's OK to have one sugary treat, such as cake *or* ice cream. Encourage him to eat this slowly, savoring every bite.
- Suggest that your child have water, 100 percent juice (1 cup maximum), or milk instead of sugar-sweetened soda.

Featured Activity: The Family Outing
Take a fun, physically active family outing.

- Go to the beach.
- Go to an amusement park.
- Go to a water park.
- Go canoeing on a lake.
- Go skiing.
- Take a day hike.
- Take a camping trip.

The Steps
- *Step Up:* Choose any Step Up goal that you didn't achieve (or want to repeat) from any week of the program.
- *Step Down:* Choose any Step Down goal that you didn't achieve (or want to repeat) from any week of the program.

Monitoring
Keep daily record of:

- Step Up goal
- Step Down goal

Rewards
- Achieving Step Up goal — 1 Program Point
- Achieving Step Down goal — 1 Program Point
- BONUS for parents for organizing family outing — kids make parents breakfast in bed

Support: Reinforcement

Negative reinforcement gets children to stop doing something out of fear of unpleasant consequences. Positive reinforcement teaches children what to do in an environment that strengthens the parent-child relationship. This week, use negative reinforcement such as nagging or punishment only when absolutely necessary; use positive reinforcement such as praise frequently. If you catch your child doing something right, tell her about it. It's also time to cash in any unused Program Points for rewards.

Tip: Come Again Soon

Return to the 9-Week Program, in whole or in part, whenever your family needs a refresher.

PART IV

Making Peace Around Us

8

CHANGING THE WORLD

By now, you're well on your way to winning the food fight with two of the three key strategies: developing eating and activity habits that quiet the battle between mind and metabolism (part II) and supporting the family as the last bastion of protection for our children (part III). But let's not stop there. The war will continue to rage as long as schools sell junk food to students, food commercials manipulate young minds, parking lots replace playgrounds, and politics puts short-term profit over our children's well-being.

Having first directed our energy within the family, let's now turn our attention outward, to make schools, communities, and the entire country a healthier place to live. In this chapter, we highlight five ordinary people — a mother, a student, a physical education (PE) teacher, a librarian, and a principal — who are doing extraordinary things to change the world. Here are their stories, in their own words.

A Mother

*Nancy Huehnergarth, the mother of two daughters ages eleven and thir-
teen, lives in a suburb of New York City. Over the past five years, she has
struggled to improve the quality of the food in her children's school district
against tremendous resistance. Along the way, she acquired the unusual distinction of being "fired from a volunteer job." Despite the obstacles, her efforts are benefiting student health throughout the state.*

In 2001, my family moved to a small suburban town in large part
because the town schools had a reputation for academic excellence.
However, a few months after my children started school, I couldn't
help but notice that the middle school cafeteria was lined with vending
machines serving every kind of junk food imaginable — candy, ice
cream, soda, chips, cookies, and so on. That wasn't right, I thought, so
I wrote a position paper on why we should have healthier foods in our
vending machines. I gave it to the PTA, which put me in touch with
other parents who felt the same way I did. We formed the PTA Nutrition Committee, and our first order of business was to improve the
content of the middle school vending machines.

Oh, how naive I was! I figured that our school leaders would read
our well-researched position paper, meet with us, and make the necessary changes. After all, we all wanted what was best for our kids,
right? But senior school leaders refused to meet with us. We were
told that our committee couldn't present our paper to the school board.
I started to hear from friends that PTA higher-ups were calling us
wackos who would stop at nothing less than removing cupcakes from
birthday parties. None of these accusations could be further from the
truth. In reality, we were a thoughtful, moderate group of parents
who simply wanted to begin a discussion about improving school food
for our children's sake. Our ideas were mainstream: adding healthy
snacks to vending machines, increasing the availability of whole grains
and fresh fruits and vegetables, and ending the practice of rewarding

children with sweets and treats in the classroom. But I continued to hear that we were being described as radical.

At this point, a number of parents dropped out of the committee. They felt they were being demonized by the school administration and were fearful about the impact on their children. One of them went back to work on Wall Street, stating, among other reasons, that a full-time job there would certainly be easier than trying to reason with district leaders! But many of us forged on, vowing to build personal relationships with school administrators, board members, and PTA leaders. We would simply have to educate them about nutrition and win them over, we reasoned.

To help inform the broader school community, we sponsored several food and nutrition events. We had Healthy Heart Week in our school cafeterias, where parents gave out samples of healthy foods to kids. We surveyed kids about what they wanted our cafeterias to serve and held seminars for parents that featured local doctors and nutrition professionals answering questions about children's nutrition issues. We also placed articles in many school publications describing the link between what kids eat and their school performance, behavior, and long-term health.

Our tenacity paid off, at least at first. We didn't go away, and the district began to react. They removed most of the offending vending machines from our middle school. The fare that remained was not perfect, but it was a vast improvement — baked chips, bottled water, pretzels, and granola bars were now the mainstays. Then we tackled beverages in the cafeterias. Our food service provider agreed to sell only water, milk, seltzer, and 100 percent fruit juice at the middle school and water, milk, and 100 percent fruit juice in the elementary schools. High school fare remained the same, but we were happy with the changes made on other levels and decided to be satisfied with small steps.

After our initial success, the group began to advocate for the creation of a district Wellness Committee that would examine school food and school food policy and make recommendations for improvement. Not surprisingly, our school leaders seemed uninterested. That changed in the fall of 2004, when a federal mandate required all schools participating in the National School Lunch Program to form a Wellness Committee and create a school wellness policy by June 2006. Our school leaders announced that they were forming a district-wide Wellness Committee and asked me to serve as a parent representative.

The first meeting took place in January 2005. It was a great meeting — well attended and focused. I left feeling encouraged. But the next scheduled meeting in February was canceled due to snow and never rescheduled, and when I showed up at the March meeting, I discovered only two other committee members in attendance. As the April meeting drew near, I wasn't feeling optimistic. Sure enough, I received an e-mail notifying the committee that the meeting had been canceled because not enough members could make it.

So here we were, four months into our new Wellness Committee mandate, with nothing to show for it. After an e-mail exchange with a co-chair which I didn't find reassuring, I felt it was time for more aggressive action. By this point, I had compiled an e-mail list of more than two hundred district parents who were interested in nutrition and school food issues. I wrote to them explaining my great disappointment with the Wellness Committee's lack of progress and asked them to contact the school board and senior administrators by e-mail. Apparently, they did so — in droves.

The outpouring from parents seemed to spur the school district to act. They scheduled an immediate meeting of the Wellness Committee and added new members. In May and June, we had three productive meetings and created standards for our cafeteria snacks and beverages that were approved by the school board during summer recess. Progress at last!

When fall arrived, however, I saw the Wellness Committee falling back into the same frustrating pattern. The first meeting was rescheduled. The second meeting was sparsely attended. At the third meeting, our co-chair arrived late and left early, and failed to bring the materials we needed. Once again, I was getting the impression that nutrition, and its effects on our children, was a very low priority.

I wrote a candid letter to the committee, the school board, and the school administration outlining missed meetings, poor attendance, lack of interest, and failure to move forward — with a June 2006 federal deadline looming. The reaction of the school administration? The superintendent asked me to step down. So there it is — I was fired from a volunteer job.

As sad as this outcome was, it turned out to be positive in many ways. No longer a member of the district team, I was now able to work outside the system. I took the issue to a *New York Times* writer who published a story about school food quality on the front page of our county's edition. That got a lot of attention. I also helped form a coalition with other interested parents, which organized a sold-out conference for school leaders interested in improving food and fitness in their districts. Representatives from forty school districts attended. Ironically, senior administrators in neighboring school districts have contacted me asking for my advice and assistance in creating better school food programs.

As far as my school district is concerned, I haven't seen much positive change in our cafeterias since I was asked to step down. Our wellness policy, as written and adapted, was deeply disappointing to many — brief and general. I don't believe it will have any real impact on what's served in our cafeterias or vending machines. There is one bright spot, however: the policy does end the practice of teachers and coaches rewarding children with candy. Baby steps!

Obviously, I feel pretty strongly about this issue. Why? For one, I fear for our children's well-being in light of the alarming medical data about their deteriorating health. I also saw my own children's eating habits adversely affected by the environment in their school. In my opinion, schools must model good nutritional habits in their cafeterias and classrooms to reinforce the lessons taught at home and in health class. And lastly, I was incensed by the dismissive way our PTA Nutrition Committee seemed to be treated from the get-go.

I plan on continuing to advocate for better school food via a state-wide alliance I'm now creating. Seeing how difficult it has been in my own district, which is blessed with resources, I'm now convinced that legislation will be the key to getting all school districts to improve.

As for my children, at first they were a bit embarrassed that their mother was leading the charge for healthy food at school. But now they appreciate my advocacy, particularly when a parent, student, or teacher thanks me for taking on this issue. And many do!

Improving school food is not easy. Too many school districts are highly resistant, either because junk food brings in needed revenue or because school leaders fail to accept that nutrition can impact the life of a child. Either way, it's going to take the continued efforts of tenacious parents to turn the tide. We don't really have a choice. Our kids are depending on us.

A Student

Eighteen-year-old Arielle Carpenter is a high school senior in Boca Raton, Florida. She began a campaign to educate her peers about health and nutrition in 2002. Her efforts have been featured in a Connect with Kids *episode called "The Biggest Generation" and she has also appeared on CNN Headline News. After finishing high school, Arielle will attend college at Tufts University, where she plans to study nutrition and public health.*

My story begins about four years ago when I started high school. About 2,500 students would eat lunch in a twenty-five-minute period. It was easier to grab a soda and chips from the vending machines in the courtyard than wait in a long line for a hot lunch in the cafeteria. Besides, most kids preferred to eat in the courtyard. I saw this going on day after day and grew concerned. I realized I wanted to do something.

I started a grass-roots campaign by contacting the Palm Beach County school superintendent, who directed me to the district's Food Service Menu Committee. They invited me to one of their planning meetings to talk about what could be done to improve school nutrition. I sat at a discussion table with the Palm Beach County school cafeteria managers and their directors. I suggested that they consider selling their prepackaged salads outside in the courtyard where they would reach more students. Unfortunately, nothing worked out. A wireless cash register system couldn't be set up in the courtyard, the salads had to be kept at an exact temperature, and they couldn't find coolers that met the specifications. They just couldn't overcome any of the regulations.

So I decided to focus my efforts elsewhere. I met with the school principal to try to convince her to at least put some healthier alternatives into the vending machines. They were filled with candy bars, greasy potato chips, and something called a "honey bun." This is basically just a big doughnut, and it was one of the most popular items. The principal said that the large profits gained from the school's vending machines would not allow them to sacrifice the money for healthier foods. But I did some research and found many studies showing that vending sales do not suffer in the long run if healthier foods are substituted. And the profits schools make from soda and vending machines are minimal in comparison to the costs of health care later on due to obesity.

After being turned down by the county and the school administration, I started doing things on my own. For FCAT (Florida Comprehensive Assessment Test) testing, students were originally going to be given processed white bagels, a food that quickly turns into sugar in the body and that might actually make students tired instead of giving them a long-lasting boost. I contacted food manufacturers directly and arranged to provide protein energy bars and drinks donated by healthy food companies. I was basically doing this on my own time. My mom helped by making the initial contact with the companies, and then I'd explain what I was doing.

After my sophomore year, I transferred to a private high school in Fort Lauderdale. This school offered all of its students a nutritious lunch, and there was also a salad bar. But after taking one look in the on-campus school store, which sold candy, soda, and chips, I felt that I still had work to do. I began by giving nutrition talks to the younger students. They were very receptive and asked lots of good questions.

I focused my presentation on the importance of making healthy food choices through balance and moderation. You don't have to eliminate candy and sweets, just eat them sparingly. I also told students how important it is to read food labels and eat breakfast, and I encouraged them to cut back on sugar. One exercise they really enjoyed is a math problem called the "soda count." You calculate how much sugar is consumed in a year if you drink just one twelve-ounce can of soda a day. When I hold up a forty-pound bag of sugar to show them the answer, I can see from their faces that I have made an impact. When I later made a presentation to the school's Mothers' Club, I learned that one boy had gone home and told his mother that he didn't want to drink soda at dinner anymore!

I've spoken to other groups in my community, such as Teen Cabaret, a place where students showcase their singing, dancing, and musical acts. I set up a nutrition table at intermission to educate students from around the area. I've also spoken to the Boca Raton Public Library Teen Advisory Board. This was an interesting experience because students come to the meeting with the promise of getting chips and candy. As I gave my presentation, I spotted them looking at the labels on the foods they were eating. They asked great questions and told their supervisor at the end to buy healthier foods next time. When asked what they wanted, they suggested things such as grapes, carrot sticks, and dried fruit. I also talked at the Rotary Youth Leadership Association three-day conference for student leaders.

I wouldn't call myself an expert. The things I talk about are pretty basic, things my mom has taught me. To me, it's common sense. But people don't seem to know that drinking soda every day isn't good for you. What bothers me most is that this is hitting my generation really hard. There are kids who are going to get very sick from being obese. I get frustrated when I see overweight children eating junk food. But I know it's not always their fault. I believe they just don't know better.

WHEN RESEARCH ISN'T FIT
FOR CONSUMPTION

❖ It's widely recognized that when a drug company pays for a research study, the results are likely to be favorable to the company's financial interests. But this issue hadn't been examined in the area of nutrition. Whereas conflicts of interest in pharmaceutical research could affect millions of patients who take medicines, conflicts of interest in nutrition research could affect everyone's health, because everyone eats.

For this reason, we examined scientific articles published over a five-year period relating to the health effects of milk, fruit juice, and soft drinks. We focused on these beverages because they are highly profitable and heavily advertised to children. To do our study fairly, one group of investigators categorized the conclusions of published articles without knowledge of the sponsorship. A second group categorized sponsorship without knowledge of the conclusions.

We found that articles supported by the food industry are almost eight times more likely to be favorable to the industry's financial interests than are articles with independent support. These findings suggest that conflicts of interest could produce extensive bias in the scientific literature, with a huge potential impact on public health. Biased science could influence government dietary guidelines, health care providers' advice to patients, and FDA regulation of food advertising claims.

Ultimately, the solution to this problem is to increase government and other independent funding of nutrition research in order to dilute any bias resulting from industry funding. In the meantime, my advice about research is to read the ingredients. If the study is paid for by industry, it may have less to do with science and more to do with marketing.

They haven't been properly educated about nutrition or healthy eating choices, either in school or at home. They've also been influenced by media marketing of fast food and snacks that are convenient and cheap. It takes work and effort to eat healthy foods. I understand this. I'm frequently faced with difficult food choices when I'm out with friends or traveling and want something quick and healthy to eat.

We cannot ignore this problem and hope it will go away. My generation may not be old enough to vote in an election, but I want them to vote with their forks!

A PE Teacher

Patty Nolan works at Warren Point Elementary School in Fair Lawn, New Jersey. She has seen a rapid increase in the number of overweight children in recent years. In response, she launched a novel health and fitness program involving the entire school. Since the program began in 2003, it has been incorporated into the curriculum of every elementary school in the district and has won a state award.

After fourteen years of teaching physical education, I began to notice an alarming trend: potbellies on elementary school students. Kids weren't playing as much as they used to, and their eating habits were terrible. As a physical education teacher, I knew there had to be something I could do.

I looked around the community. My PTA was coming up with some plans of its own to address childhood obesity. The group had talked about starting a health and fitness program at one of their first meetings, but their efforts seemed to be stagnating. Although they were willing to fund a program, there was no leadership to make it happen. The school principal was in his fifteenth year. He was a very good principal and very connected, but he had his hands full. I knew there was no way for him to institute a new program without major help.

One of my duties was to patrol the lunchroom, which was also the gymnasium. I saw so much junk going into kids' mouths. There was candy, soda, Ring Dings, Yodels, Double Stuff Oreos — you name the junk food, and the kids were eating it. It was disheartening, and I didn't want to watch passively as kids ate this stuff and grew fatter. When I first started teaching, I never noticed much obesity. Now I would say half the kids are becoming obese. You can see it when they're in physical education class: they're uncomfortable, they get tired quickly, and they have to take breaks more often. If they don't change their lifestyles at a young age, they're just going to grow heavier and heavier and suffer from many health problems as adults. But to make a difference, they need to do more than take a weekly physical education class.

So I called a meeting to pick up where the PTA health and fitness idea had left off. The meeting was well attended. There were moms from all grade levels, a few teachers, and the school nurse. There were students, too. Everyone was really enthusiastic about doing something to make kids healthier. The meeting ended after thirty minutes with parents walking out of the room with various assignments. I had a lot of professionals to tap into: a salesperson, a writer, and individuals with connections to healthy foods. Everyone had ideas, and things really started happening from there.

My main focus was to get the community moving. The plan we came up with had three different layers. First, find activities that most kids would like. Second, get parents involved — kids are more likely to be active if they see their parents moving. Third, put together a large event that involved the whole community. I knew that we needed a reward system to motivate the kids to move. There were so many things to think about.

I started by getting kids involved at lunchtime. Every lunch period, every day of the week, a different fitness activity takes place. On Moving Mondays, I run laps around the school grounds with the kids, cheering them on. The math teachers encourage children to log their miles and add up their results. Tournament Tuesdays have competitive games between teams; 85 percent of the students participate, and final winners earn awards at lunch. On Walkin' & Wheelin' Wednesdays, kids and parents walk, Rollerblade, or bike to school. Once kids do this fifteen times, they get on the health and fitness honor roll. On Thirsty Thursdays, everyone brings a water bottle to school and learns the benefits of staying hydrated. I've heard that at home, kids are more often taking a water bottle out of the refrigerator instead of a soda. On Fat Free Fridays, healthy eating is encouraged, and the school doesn't sell ice cream or unhealthy snacks during lunch. Kids accept it and don't complain. It's just become part of the routine.

Since the program started, the kids have been really excited about competing in tournaments, running laps, and promoting healthy eating. Just about every student in the school has participated. And with the parents signing permission slips, they're aware of the revolution going on during lunch hour.

Other aspects of the program are academic. We had a contest in which every student drew a picture or wrote an essay about eating healthy. One year, we had a poster and motto contest. The winning slogan was "Get Fit, Don't Quit."

The first year, we also held a fitness expo for the school community. We had healthy food donations and several twenty- to thirty-minute time periods filled with different exercises: stretching, kickboxing, strength training, and line dancing. Dentists and chiropractors lectured students and parents about healthy habits, and massage therapists offered ten-minute neck and shoulder rubs for relaxation. It was truly a fantastic event with a very high level of participation.

Another event that has continued annually is the run/walk involving families throughout the community. The event requires the local police to block off streets, letters to be distributed to each affected household near the school, and several planning meetings with parents and staff. Early in the morning, we set up signs for the route and tables for donated food and water. First graders do one lap around the route (equal to one mile); second and third graders do two laps, and fourth and fifth graders do three laps. Everyone who passes the finish line is a winner and gets a medal. There is no first place or last place. The first year, we were fortunate to get the help of a parent DJ who spun popular tunes on his awesome sound system, and he continues to play for us every year. We have prizes for everyone.

Year after year, the response to the program has been overwhelmingly great. Kids have started bringing healthy treats for birthdays — peanut butter and apple slices, carrots, broccoli. Parents have really gotten into it, too. Some have scooped out a watermelon and used the shell as a bowl for fruit salad. The kids come to the gym to show me their healthy birthday treats. They are so proud of themselves.

Money has been a factor throughout. I receive only $1,500 annually from the school but have been able to get private donations. Any money left over is put toward workout equipment for the school or used to help fund a new playground.

The experience of organizing and overseeing this program has taught me a lot about leadership. I'm a planner and a facilitator, and I can get people excited to do things. It's rewarding to hear comments from the kids, for example, when they ask if they can still run on Mondays even if it rains. Parents tell me they're walking more, watching what they eat, and losing weight. The kids are starting to eat better, to get more exercise, and to do it as a family. Self-esteem is building. As for the future, I know wherever I go and wherever I work, health and fitness will be a priority.

A Librarian

Teresa Garceau works at the Calvin Leete Elementary School in Guilford, Connecticut. In 2003, she created a course on the media for third and fourth graders. The students learn about methods used by advertising agencies to sell junk food to kids and then make commercials for healthy foods that air on local TV. The course has become wildly popular with students and parents.

As a librarian, I've noticed more and more significantly overweight children entering school each year. Recently, one class of thirteen had six kids who were heavy. Once, I recall seeing a child about 50 pounds overweight enter the school holding hands with his mother, who weighed about 250 pounds. Three of his classmates were giggling, making derogatory references to Jell-O. It was heartbreaking. I felt like telling those kids that all children are special and we should treat others the way we want them to treat us. This kind of teasing happened a lot, but not wanting to offend anyone, I felt I had few options available to deal with these situations. Then I realized that as a media specialist, I had the perfect opportunity to educate children with information about the benefits of health, physical exercise, and nutrition.

I considered my own family. In our fifties, my husband and I run and work out almost every day. We have raised three children who are conscious of what they eat and have reaped the benefits of being physically active. Our oldest son played Division I hockey for West Point. Our second son will be playing on West Point's lacrosse team next year. Our daughter was a figure skater with a synchronized skating team that achieved ninth place at the world competition in Milan in 2003.

We believe that our children's healthy habits began with our own efforts to learn about good nutrition and model these behaviors for them. They grew to understand the importance of a nutritious breakfast (we had lots of oatmeal). Homemade soups were frequently served. I didn't buy junk food or processed foods, and I served few high-calorie desserts. To this day, we don't crave them.

So I decided to develop a course, in collaboration with the teachers, with the goal of educating the students about healthy eating and physical activity. However, my first attempts didn't succeed. We focused too much on academics, and the kids got bored. In an effort to make things more interesting the second year, I began to brainstorm with one of my parent volunteers, and we came up with a concept that made us burst with excitement. Children see thousands of TV commercials each year. We decided to teach them about how commercials are made and have them make one themselves.

Together with the teachers, we began the research phase of the project. The first assignment was for the students to spend a weekend watching children's programming and write down what they noticed about advertisements. How many commercials were about food? How do advertisers get kids excited about their products? We listed all the strategies, such as using popular celebrities, making exaggerated claims about nutrition, constantly repeating things, using catchy tunes, and offering free toys.

Next, we divided the classes into groups of four or five. Each group had to choose one item from the Food Guide Pyramid and make a commercial to persuade people to eat it. I was astounded at the results that the third and fourth graders came up with! We had antioxidants dressed up as blueberries with swords, fighting free radicals, and lawyers making the case for fraud by citing the ingredients listed on boxes of sugary cereal. The health effects of soda were shown in a sugar count, and trans fats were exposed as the villains that they are. Kids posed as chefs, gym teachers, and TV anchors with late-breaking stories warning about the hazards of junk food. Everyone in the school knew about the commercials being produced in the library.

Very soon, the students began to realize that not all foods are nutritionally equal. It was a teacher's dream to observe their creativity, critical thinking, enthusiasm, and teamwork. The kids taught each other and became so excited to see each other's productions. One of our fourth graders said that the experience made him "think about what goes into my mouth" instead of just eating. He is now aware that the commercials are trying to get his money, and he realizes that healthy choices are better for his body. We're adopting techniques that Madison Avenue uses against children and fighting back.

Finally, we produced the commercials using iMovie and a digital camera, and we added a music overlay. (Any moviemaking program will work.) My parent volunteer loved helping the kids with the production and editing. The finished commercials were aired on GCTV, a community access channel.

Learning how to care for their bodies should be a vital part of children's education today. I feel enthusiastic about continuing this project. I love what I do, and I live it!

A Principal

Oliver Barton helped create a charter high school in New Haven, Connecticut, that is also a working farm. At this innovative school, students pursue traditional studies while developing a deep understanding of the connections between food production, health, and the environment.

I first became interested in working with teenagers on health and fitness issues in the 1980s as a young teacher in an urban public school in Connecticut. I saw so many students who ate extremely poorly — a bag of chips and a large soda for breakfast as just one example. And many of these students seemed to be completely apathetic about physical and mental challenges throughout the day. I remembered having a similar experience in middle school, being a bit overweight and not very athletic and feeling disconnected. Although my family tried to provide healthier foods, it wasn't until high school that I became committed to physical activity and motivated to get in shape.

So I decided that something should be done about this situation. I started taking kids backpacking and found other programs that could challenge them and instill pride and confidence. I co-taught a high school class that met at a local nature center. Students studied ecology, grew food, heated the classroom with a woodstove, and discussed how their personal choices influenced them and the global environment. They were fascinated with learning how their bodies worked and became interested in nutrition as they grew food and prepared it. It turned out that studying about their bodies and nutrition helped interest the teenagers in health and science. As we developed that course and others, such as the politics of food, students began to see connections between the local food environment and issues around the world.

In 1990, a local activist and I discussed the idea of having a whole high school with an environmental theme and an organic farm. The idea was to tap kids' innate interest in food and the natural environment and provide a challenging academic setting as well. We involved others and started a nonprofit organization, the New Haven Ecology Project. We also developed several pilot programs, such as teacher training, service learning clubs, and a summer camp. When Connecticut first authorized the creation of charter schools, we submitted a proposal, received approval, and set up Common Ground High School on twenty acres of undeveloped land leased from the city.

Since then, Common Ground has grown into a unique learning environment where students can explore a range of issues relating to the food supply, ecology, politics, and community service, all while developing hands-on experience in the operation of a working farm. In addition to their academic studies, students participate in growing six to eight tons of produce per year. They help sell the food at farmers' markets and to a local restaurant, and they help prepare it for donation to local soup kitchens. Each day, our school lunch offers students a nutritious selection of whole foods. We have no vending machines and provide healthier snacks for free.

The farm hosts programs for families on weekends (such as free "pick your own" days), workshops for adults in the evening, farm festivals, and a summer camp. All this is very far from what students are used to. At first the kids are often shocked by the source of their food. They say, "I'm not eating carrots that come out of the dirt" or "I don't eat eggs that come out of chickens." But after helping to grow and cook food, their tastes mature, and students can be heard complaining if there is no fresh green salad. Many, eager to get in shape, can be seen choosing a healthy light lunch every day. After a while, they become less winded when they walk up the steep driveway to the school. Although not every student experiences a dramatic transformation of health habits, everyone, I believe, thinks seriously at some point about what they are used to eating, where it comes from, and how it affects them.

Many scientists now believe that this is the first generation of young people who will have a shorter life expectancy than their parents due to lack of exercise and poor diet. Parents and citizens concerned about health around the country are taking on state legislatures, school districts, and individual schools to surround kids with healthier options. Research in Connecticut shows that such actions make a difference. My firsthand experience has shown me that the local food environment and how we encourage healthy activity and food choices make a big difference. Spend a few days seeing the world from a child's perspective: What food is available? What's tempting? Are there healthier choices within sight? Ask what most kids eat at school and why. Speak with others who are concerned; get advice from nurses, doctors, and books; and consider your own experience growing up. You'll be armed with enough information and outrage to talk to others and raise questions, discuss possible changes, and expect results at your local schools and even area businesses. Through these actions, we can change the food environment and help reverse the trend of declining health that affects everyone in our communities.

PART V

Increase the Peace

9

RECIPES

Anchor Your Day with Breakfast

You've heard it before — breakfast is the most important meal of the day. And yet it has become the most commonly skipped meal of the day as well.

Of all the times you might feel "starving" for something to eat, this is the time you actually are. After fasting for eight to twelve hours or more, your body is running on empty and needs a boost of energy to keep things running smoothly. Muscles need fuel for the physical activities of the day, and the brain needs fuel to keep you concentrating and thinking clearly.

Besides, skipping breakfast invariably leads to overeating later in the day: by afternoon, your body will be screaming for food. To satisfy that overwhelming hunger, you'll most likely blow right past the point of "pleasantly full" and barrel headlong into "overstuffed." Like a car, your body requires a steady, constant supply of fuel, and breakfast is the most important time to provide it.

The following breakfast recipes combine whole grains, fruits and vegetables, and protein in tasty combinations to anchor your day. Some of the recipes, such as Breakfast Burrito (page 220), can be taken out the door. Others, such as Whole Wheat Pancakes (page 221) and The Omelet Classic (page 213), are more traditional, sit-down breakfast foods.

The quickest option is store-bought cereal, and the guidelines in the QUICK PICK! Store-Bought Cold Cereal recipe below will help you make the best choices. (Look for other QUICK PICK! recipes throughout this chapter.)

Enjoy a healthy breakfast to start a great day.

QUICK PICK!

❖ Store-Bought Cold Cereal

Cold cereal can be part of a healthy breakfast. However, many store-bought cereals are the nutritional equivalent of a bowl of sugar. When choosing a cereal, look at the label to see if it meets the following three criteria, or try making your own cold cereal (see Muesli, page 207).

1. Whole grains are listed as the first ingredient.
2. Sugar (or any of its relatives, such as high-fructose corn syrup) is *not* listed as one of the first two ingredients.
3. A serving provides at least 4 grams of fiber.

Some widely available brands that fit this description include Kashi GoLean Crunch!, Barbara's Bakery Puffins, Post Grape-Nuts, Post Original Shredded Wheat, Familia Swiss Müesli, and Uncle Sam.

To serve: Combine 1 serving of the cereal with 1 cup low-fat milk or plain soy milk. Top off with fresh or dried fruit and nuts (optional).

❖ Muesli

Yield: Twelve ½-cup servings

Muesli (pronounced "mews-lee") is a breakfast cereal invented in the early 1900s by Maximilian Bircher-Benner, a Swiss physician and pioneer of nutritional research, who believed a diet based on grains, nuts, fruits, and vegetables could be used to heal his patients at his Zurich health center. Bircher-Benner's muesli recipe combined oats, lemon juice, condensed milk, apples, and nuts, but you can now find many versions of muesli described in cookbooks and available as prepackaged cereals. The guiding principle, however, remains the same: combine whole grains, fruits, and nuts with healthier dairy products for a nutrient-rich start to your day.

A quick trip to your local natural food store's bulk foods section will give you the largest choice of whole grain flakes — oat, wheat, rye, barley, and more. These are whole grains that have been rolled into flat flakes (like the oats used to make oatmeal). The best part about this recipe is that it is absolutely foolproof. Can't find rye flakes? Just use more of the wheat flakes — or try wheat bran or wheat germ. Tired of almonds? Substitute walnuts, pecans, hazelnuts, or a combination of the three. Add a tablespoon of sesame seeds, sunflower seeds, or pumpkin seeds. Or substitute dried blueberries or other dried fruit for the raisins. Gather your family around and create your very own breakfast cereal.

2½ cups rolled oats (not instant or quick-cooking)
1 cup chopped raw almonds
½ cup wheat flakes
½ cup rye flakes
½ cup barley flakes
1 cup raisins or dried currants

Low-fat milk or plain low-fat yogurt, for serving

Fresh berries, grated apple, or pure maple syrup (optional), for
serving

Preheat the oven to 350 degrees F.

In a large roasting pan, add the rolled oats, almonds, wheat flakes,
rye flakes, and barley flakes. Stir to combine.

Bake, stirring occasionally, until the oats just begin to take on a bit
of golden color, 5 to 7 minutes. Let cool; stir in the raisins. Transfer the
mixture to an airtight container and store at room temperature for up
to 2 months.

To serve, combine ½ cup muesli with ½ cup milk (cold or hot) or
plain low-fat yogurt. If you like, you can add a sprinkling of fresh berries or grated apple or a teaspoon of maple syrup for sweetness.

❖ Steel-Cut Oats

Yield: Four 1-cup servings

If you think oatmeal means tearing open a little packet of pulverized
oat flakes and adding boiling water, you haven't had steel-cut oats. Instant oatmeal is refined, processed, and treated for instant cooking —
which also results in instant digestion. Steel-cut oats are the whole
grain groats (or the inner portion of the oat kernel) that have been cut,
not rolled and pounded, into just two or three pieces. Steel-cut oats
take longer to cook but maintain their oat structure, which slows
down their digestion and keeps your blood sugar stable for hours.
These are the oats that Grandma called her "stick to your ribs" breakfast. With the following methods, there is no reason you can't have a
bowl of hot steel-cut oats whenever you want one. Try topping a bowl
with fresh fruit, toasted nuts, a drizzle of maple syrup, or a swirl of all-
fruit preserves.

4 cups water

Pinch of salt

1 cup steel-cut oats (not rolled, quick-cooking, or instant)

Your favorite topping (see page 210), for serving

Eat Now Method: Bring the water to a boil in a medium saucepan. Add the salt and slowly stir the oats into the boiling water. Return to a boil; immediately reduce the heat and simmer, stirring often, until thick and creamy, 20 to 30 minutes — a little less time for chewier oats, a little more time for creamier results. Serve hot with your favorite topping.

Eat Tomorrow Method: Just before bedtime, bring the water to a boil in a medium saucepan. Add the salt and slowly stir the oats into the boiling water. Cover the pan and remove from the heat. Let sit at room temperature overnight.

When ready to eat, remove the cover and bring the oats back to a boil over high heat, stirring often. Immediately reduce the heat and simmer, stirring often, until thick and creamy, 8 to 10 minutes. Serve hot with your favorite topping.

Eat in the Next Day or Two Method: Cook the oats according to either of the previous two methods. Transfer to a medium microwave-safe container or divide among four 1-cup microwave-safe containers. Let cool to room temperature before covering. Refrigerate. (The oats will keep, refrigerated, for at least a few days.)

To serve, reheat the oats, uncovered, in the microwave for 2 minutes on high. If the oats are too thick for your taste, add a bit of water or milk and stir. Heat for another 1 to 2 minutes, or until hot. Serve with your favorite topping.

Alternatively, combine the oats and 2 to 3 tablespoons water in a small saucepan. Heat over medium heat, stirring often, until hot, about 5 minutes. Serve with your favorite topping.

A WEEK'S WORTH OF TOPPINGS
FOR STEEL-CUT OATS

❖ Here are a variety of toppings to guarantee that you'll never have a boring breakfast. Toast some nuts (see page 211) and store in an airtight container. Try ground cinnamon, cardamom, nutmeg, pumpkin pie spice, and other "sweet" spices that can trick your palate into skipping the sugar. A dash of vanilla extract or almond extract can do the same. A small handful of dried fruit stirred into your oats is lovely on a winter morning. And if you need something sweeter every now and then, all-fruit preserves, maple syrup, honey, and agave nectar (see page 223) are fine in small drizzles.

Monday: 1 tablespoon chopped toasted nuts and a dusting of ground cinnamon

Tuesday: A teaspoon or two of all-fruit preserves stirred into the oats with or without ½ cup low-fat milk or vanilla soy milk

Wednesday: A small handful of fresh strawberries (or other fresh fruit), sliced, with or without ½ cup low-fat milk or vanilla soy milk

Thursday: 1 tablespoon chopped toasted nuts, 1 tablespoon chopped dried fruit (apricots, apples, sour cherries, blueberries), and a dusting of ground cinnamon

Friday: 1 tablespoon peanut butter (thinned with 1 tablespoon very hot water) swirled into the oats with 1 tablespoon jam or preserves

Saturday: 2 tablespoons fresh berries and 1 tablespoon granola for a bit of crunch

Sunday: 2 tablespoons low-fat yogurt and a sprinkling of granola

Eat Anytime This Month Method: Cook the oats according to either of the first two methods. Divide the cooked oats among four 1-cup freezer-safe containers. Let cool to room temperature before covering. Place in the freezer. (The oats will keep, frozen, for up to 1 month.)

TOASTING NUTS

❖ Toasting nuts in the oven makes them taste more "nutty" reduces any bitterness. To preserve even more of their flavor, toast nuts whole and chop them just before using.

Preheat the oven to 350 degrees F. Spread the nuts on a rimmed baking sheet or in a very shallow baking dish. Place in the oven, stirring occasionally and watching constantly, until fragrant and lightly browned:

- 5 to 10 minutes for almonds and pecans
- 8 to 10 minutes for walnuts
- 10 to 12 minutes for hazelnuts

Watch carefully, as nuts can go from toasted to burned very quickly.

Let cool. Store in an airtight container at room temperature for up to 2 weeks.

Note: The "puck" that forms when you freeze the oatmeal can be transferred to a large resealable plastic bag if you don't want to tie up your freezer-safe containers. You can also freeze the cooked oatmeal in a plastic ice cube tray, then transfer the cubes to a large resealable plastic bag. You'll want to reheat 3 or 4 cubes for breakfast, depending on the size of your cubes.

To serve, reheat the frozen oats, uncovered, in a microwave-safe container in the microwave for 2 to 3 minutes on high. If the oats are too thick for your taste, add a bit of water or milk and stir. Heat for another 1 to 2 minutes, or until hot. Serve with your favorite topping.

Alternatively, defrost the frozen oats, then combine them with 2 to 3 tablespoons water in a small saucepan. Heat over medium heat, stirring often, until hot, about 5 minutes. Serve with your favorite topping.

❖ Hot Brown Rice Breakfast Porridge

Yield: Four ½-cup servings

Porridge is made in many cultures around the world by boiling oats, rice, or other grains in water or milk until they reach the consistency of a thick, creamy pudding. The Irish and the Scots cook oat groats in milk, the Chinese make *jook* (also called *congee*) with rice and water, and the Finns enjoy *ruishiutaleita,* or "rye porridge," for breakfast.

You can take a bit of cooked brown rice left over from last night's dinner and combine it with vanilla soy milk or regular milk, a little protein powder, and a pinch of salt to make a warm, creamy, satisfying breakfast — and you get the benefit of whole grain nutrition first thing in the morning. If you haven't used soy milk before, this is the perfect time to try it.

1½ cups vanilla soy milk, regular soy milk plus ½ teaspoon
    vanilla extract, or low-fat milk plus ½ teaspoon vanilla
    extract
1 tablespoon soy protein powder (optional)
Pinch of salt
1 cup cooked brown rice

Toppings (optional)
Ground cinnamon
Finely chopped toasted nuts (see page 211)
Finely chopped dried fruit

In a medium saucepan, whisk together the soy milk, protein powder, and salt until the protein powder has dissolved. Add the rice and stir to combine. Bring to a boil over medium-high heat. Reduce the heat to low and simmer, stirring occasionally, until almost all of the milk has been absorbed, about 15 minutes. Remove from the heat, cover, and let sit for 5 minutes.

Serve hot with the toppings of your choice, if desired.

❖ The Omelet Classic

Yield: 1 serving

Find the freshest eggs, grind your own pepper, and turn up the heat. Omelets are made in a flash — and fillings are limited only by your imagination. Use Mix-and-Match Omelet Fillings on page 214 for inspiration.

1 large egg plus 2 large egg whites, or ½ cup liquid egg substitute

1 teaspoon water

Pinch of salt

A few grinds of black pepper

½ teaspoon extra virgin olive oil or unsalted butter

¼ cup filling of your choice (see headnote)

In a small bowl, combine the eggs, water, salt, and pepper. Using a fork, whisk until combined.

Heat the olive oil or butter in an 8-inch skillet over medium-high heat. Add the egg mixture and stir with a fork until the eggs just begin to set, about 10 seconds. As the eggs continue to set, gently pull the cooked eggs into the center of the pan, tilting the pan so that the liquid eggs move to the side of the pan where they can cook more easily. Continue until the entire omelet is lightly set, 20 to 30 seconds. Let the omelet cook, undisturbed, until just barely browned on the bottom and still a bit creamy on top, about 10 seconds more. Don't let it cook too long, or you will lose the tender, creamy quality of a perfectly cooked omelet.

Spoon your choice of filling over half of the omelet. Using a spatula, flip the other half of the omelet over the filling. Carefully slide the omelet onto a plate and serve immediately.

MIX-AND-MATCH OMELET FILLINGS

❖ Very few foods *don't* make a good filling for an omelet — or topping for scrambled eggs or tofu. The French even sneak chopped apples and cinnamon inside their omelets. Plan ahead by keeping some pre-prepped, simple fillings on hand — grated cheese, leftover cooked veggies, and fresh or dried herbs. Some fillings can even be purchased ready to use — canned artichoke hearts, roasted green chiles, roasted red peppers, or frozen vegetables (defrost them first) such as spinach or chard.

MIX-AND-MATCH OMELET FILLINGS

Pick an item, or combine a few, from each column to create your very own omelet filling. Use about ¼ cup of filling per omelet.

Cheeses — coarsely grated	Vegetables — blanched, sautéed, steamed, or roasted	Flavorings
Cheddar, mild or sharp	Artichoke hearts	Basil
Cottage cheese	Asparagus	Chives
Cream cheese, low-fat	Bell peppers	Cilantro
Feta	Broccoli	Curry powder
Goat cheese	Chard	Dill
Gouda	Collards	Guacamole
Gruyère	Green onions	Marjoram
Monterey Jack	Kale	Nuts
Mozzarella	Mixed roasted veggies	Oregano
Parmesan	Mushrooms	Parsley
Pepper Jack	Mustard greens	Red pepper flakes
Ricotta	Onions (yellow or red)	Salsa
Romano	Roasted green chiles	Spaghetti or
Swiss	Roasted red peppers	pizza sauce
	Snow peas	Thyme
	Spinach	
	Tomatoes	
	Zucchini	

Note on cheese: It takes only a little cheese to get a lot of flavor.
Note on vegetables: See The Foolproof Guide to Cooking Vegetables on page 256 if you are unsure how to cook these vegetables.

❖ Curried Tofu Scramble

Yield: 4 servings

Don't be afraid: tofu might sound intimidating, but it's readily available in most grocery stores, it's easy to prepare, and best of all, it's full of high-protein nutrition. Tofu's neutral flavor makes it easy to add to almost any meal, including breakfast, as in this scramble.

You'll get perfectly scrambled tofu every time if you follow two suggestions: First, choose firm or extra-firm regular tofu (see page 216). The silken style will turn to mush and is much better suited to making sauces, dips, and smoothies (see page 224), where its ultra-creamy texture is most appreciated.

Second, drain enough water out of the tofu to give it the texture of moist scrambled eggs, but not so much that the tofu turns dry when cooked. The best way to achieve this is to break the tofu into pieces the size of an unshelled walnut, and then gently squeeze the tofu (over the sink) to remove as much water as you can without having the tofu squirt through your fingers. Place the drained tofu in a bowl and proceed with the recipe.

1½ teaspoons extra virgin olive oil
3 tablespoons minced bell pepper (red, yellow, orange, green, or a combination)
1 tablespoon minced onion
1 teaspoon minced garlic
1 teaspoon curry powder
1 pound firm or extra-firm regular tofu, drained (see headnote) and crumbled into small pieces
1 cup cooked broccoli florets, coarsely chopped
Salt and freshly ground black pepper
Chopped green onions or fresh cilantro, for garnish

Heat the olive oil in a medium skillet over medium-high heat. Add the bell pepper and onion and cook, stirring, until just tender, 2 to 3 minutes. Stir in the garlic and curry and cook until fragrant, 1 minute. Add the tofu and stir or toss gently until the tofu is lightly golden, about 2 minutes. Add the broccoli and heat through, 1 to 2 minutes. Season with salt and pepper to taste.

Transfer to a plate, garnish with green onions, and serve immediately.

A TOFU PRIMER

❖ Food historians generally believe that tofu, or bean curd, was invented in northern China sometime around 164 b.c., during the Han dynasty. But what exactly is this tofu that millions of people have been enjoying ever since?

Tofu is wonderfully versatile, flavor neutral, and high in protein. It is made by adding a special salt, such as calcium sulfate, or seaweed to soy milk, which causes curds to form (much like adding enzymes to milk to make cheese). Tofu manufacturers control taste and texture by varying how much salt (or seaweed) they use. The curds are then drained, pressed into blocks, and packaged in square plastic tubs to be sold in the refrigerator section of your grocery store.

Tofu is divided into two main kinds: regular and silken. Both kinds of tofu are further categorized by texture: soft, medium, firm, and extra-firm.

Regular tofu holds its shape well and is the best choice for stir-fries, stews, soups, and salads — when you want the tofu to hold its cubed or sliced shape. Firm or extra-firm regular tofu can be crumbled to stand in for scrambled eggs or sliced and marinated to stand in for meat. If you want to save time, look for baked tofu — regular tofu that has been flavored with a marinade and pressed into a "cake." Use it the way you would firm or extra-firm regular tofu.

Silken tofu is made with a slightly different process (more like making yogurt than making curds for cheese) resulting in a creamier, smoother, more custardy texture. Silken tofu is the best choice for making smoothies, dips, sauces, and other pureed recipes.

Tofu tastes best fresh, so check the "best used by" date and don't open the package until you are ready to use the tofu. Tofu doesn't freeze well.

Try Curried Tofu Scramble (page 215), Silky Berry-Bursting Smoothie (page 225), or Salad Bar Stir-Fry with Tofu or Chicken (page 268) for starters. Tofu makes a tasty substitute for chicken in BBQ Chicken Roll-Up (page 241), Hearty Barley, Vegetable, and Chicken Soup (page 270), or even Fajitas (page 275). Or add some to Spaghetti Veggie Medley (page 266) or Bean Chili (page 271) for a more substantial dinner.

Tofu is a master of disguise. If you don't tell, no one else will guess it's bean curd.

❖ "Sausage," Egg, and Cheese Breakfast Sandwich

Yield: 1 serving

You'll find a variety of vegetable- and/or soy-based sausage substitutes in the healthy foods section of your grocer's freezer. The patties and links are quite good as they are, but dusting them with herbs such as thyme, sage, or savory will create the more traditional "sausage" flavor. Or buy herb blends such as poultry seasoning or Italian seasoning to save time, money, and room on your spice shelf. (See more about setting up a basic spice pantry on page 227) Get the kids involved by having them cut out the rounds of bread. (They're more likely to eat healthily if they've had a hand in preparing the meal.)

2 slices sturdy whole wheat or sourdough bread
1 veggie breakfast sausage patty
Pinch of finely minced fresh thyme or dried thyme (or your
    favorite salt-free seasoning blend)

Salt and freshly ground black pepper
1 teaspoon extra virgin olive oil
1 large egg or ¼ cup liquid egg substitute
1 tablespoon grated cheddar cheese
1 thick slice ripe tomato

Using a round, 4-inch cookie cutter, cut out 2 bread circles. (You can use a regular slice of bread if you don't have a cookie cutter.) Toast the circles and set aside.

Cook the veggie sausage patty according to the package directions and season with the thyme and salt and pepper to taste. Place on one of the toasted bread circles.

Meanwhile, heat the olive oil in a small skillet over medium-high heat. In a small bowl, combine the egg and a pinch of salt and pepper. Beat with a fork until lightly scrambled. Pour the egg into the hot pan and cook, stirring occasionally, until just set, 2 to 3 minutes.

Place the egg on top of the veggie sausage patty and sprinkle with the grated cheese. Top with the tomato slice and the other toast circle and serve immediately.

❖ Cinnamon-Orange French Toast

Yield: 4 servings

The French call French toast *pain perdu,* which means "lost bread." It is the perfect way to use up day-old bread, and if you use a whole grain variety, it is a clever and tasty way to sneak some whole grains into your diet. If you'd like, top with a robustly flavored maple syrup (see more about sweeteners on page 223) or a dollop of yogurt and some sliced fruit, and you have a satisfying and healthy start to your day.

3 large eggs plus 2 large egg whites, or 1 cup liquid egg
    substitute

1⅓ cups low-fat milk or soy milk

½ teaspoon vanilla extract

½ teaspoon grated orange zest

¼ teaspoon ground cinnamon

Pinch of salt

1 teaspoon unsalted butter

1 teaspoon high-oleic safflower oil or extra virgin olive oil

8 slices hearty whole grain bread

Toppings (optional)

2 cups sliced fruit (fresh or defrosted frozen)

1 cup plain low-fat yogurt

Pure maple syrup or other sweetener

Whisk the eggs in a bowl until the yolks and whites are well blended. Add the milk, vanilla, orange zest, cinnamon, and salt. Whisk to combine.

Heat ½ teaspoon of the butter and ½ teaspoon of the oil on a griddle or in a very large skillet over medium-high heat.

In the meantime, pour the egg mixture into a large, shallow dish. (A 9-by-13-inch baking dish works very well.) Add four of the bread slices and let them soak up the egg mixture, turning them once to coat both sides evenly.

When the butter-oil mixture is hot, carefully transfer the soaked bread to the griddle and cook until golden brown, 3 to 5 minutes. Turn the slices over and cook until the other side is golden brown, 3 to 5 minutes more. Transfer to a plate and keep warm, if you like, in a 200 degree F oven while you cook the remaining French toast.

Heat the remaining butter and oil over medium-high heat. Soak and cook the remaining four slices of bread as described above.

Serve hot with the toppings of your choice, if desired.

❖ Breakfast Burrito

Yield: 1 serving

Burritos for breakfast? Why not. They're tasty and hearty, and they travel well — all characteristics that are appreciated on a busy week-day morning. Use the black beans whole, or mash half of them and leave the rest whole for a more interesting texture. Canned beans are fine; just be sure to rinse and drain them in a fine-mesh strainer before using.

> One 7- or 9-inch whole grain tortilla
> 2 tablespoons cooked black beans or vegetarian-style refried
>   beans
> 1 tablespoon grated sharp cheddar or Monterey Jack cheese
> 1 tablespoon mashed or diced avocado
> 1 teaspoon chopped green onions or minced red onion
> Shredded lettuce
> Salsa
> Chopped fresh cilantro (optional)

Heat the tortilla on a hot griddle or in a large skillet over medium heat. Heat the beans in a pot over medium heat, smashing and stirring them, until hot, 2 to 3 minutes. Put the tortilla on a plate and place the beans down the center, stopping about 2 inches short of one edge. (Alternatively, you can heat the tortilla and beans on a microwave-safe plate in the microwave on high until the beans are hot, about 1 minute.)

Top the beans with the cheese, avocado, and green onions. Add let-tuce, salsa, and cilantro (if using) to taste. Roll up burrito-style and serve hot.

❖ Whole Wheat Pancakes

Yield: About eight 4-inch pancakes

These pancakes are light, fluffy, and whole wheat. You can customize each to order with chopped apples and pecans, chopped bananas and walnuts, or blueberries and almonds. Besides the obvious topping of maple syrup, try sliced bananas, strawberries, or peaches with a dollop of plain low-fat yogurt and a sprinkling of almonds or granola. Pancakes taste best served hot off the griddle. If you want to serve them all at once, arrange them in a single layer on an ovenproof plate and place them, uncovered, in a preheated 200 degree F oven.

1 cup whole wheat flour
1 teaspoon baking powder
¼ teaspoon baking soda
Big pinch of salt
1 cup buttermilk
1 large egg or ¼ cup liquid egg substitute
1½ teaspoons pure maple syrup
1½ teaspoons melted unsalted butter or canola oil
1½ cup low-fat milk

Mix-Ins (optional)

Use ½–1 tablespoon of any of the following ingredients in combination per pancake:
• Chopped fruit: apples, bananas, peaches, pears
• Berries: blueberries, raspberries, sliced strawberries
• Chopped toasted nuts: almonds, walnuts, pecans, hazelnuts
• Chopped dried fruit: apricots, apples, peaches, raisins, figs
• Crunchy grains: granola, wheat germ, rolled oats

Pure maple syrup or your favorite topping, for serving

In a large bowl, whisk together the whole wheat flour, baking powder, baking soda, and salt. Make a small well in the center of the dry ingredients and set aside.

In a medium bowl, combine the buttermilk, egg, maple syrup, butter, and ¼ cup of the milk. Whisk until well combined.

Pour the wet ingredients into the well of the dry ingredients. Stir just until all the ingredients are combined but the mixture is still a bit lumpy. If the batter seems very stiff, thin with a bit more milk. You want ¼ cup of the batter to spread into a 4-inch pancake on the griddle.

Heat a well-seasoned griddle or large skillet over medium heat. When hot, wipe quickly with a lightly oiled paper towel or spritz (off the heat) with vegetable cooking spray. You will probably need to grease the pan only once, before the first batch of pancakes. Spoon or ladle ¼ cup of batter onto the hot griddle, leaving at least 2 inches between the pancakes. If using mix-ins, sprinkle them on the pancakes. Cook until the edges begin to set and the bottom is golden, about 2 minutes. Carefully flip the pancakes and continue to cook until the other side is golden and the centers have risen and feel a bit springy to the touch, 1 to 2 minutes more.

Serve with warm maple syrup or your favorite topping.

HOW SWEET IT IS!

❖ The debate continues as to which sweeteners are best. Although artificial sweeteners provide no calories, the jury is still out on their long-term safety when consumed in large amounts. Luckily, the "real thing" in moderation is just fine. The key is *moderation* (a teaspoon or two per serving is usually plenty) and selecting the best *natural* sweeteners available.

Maple Syrup: Seek out real (pure) maple syrup, not the maple-flavored products commonly sold. From the very light, delicate maple flavor of Grade A Light Amber to the dark, strong maple flavor of Grade B, maple syrup is a tasty sweetener for drinks, breakfast cereals, and baked goods.

Honey: There are more than three hundred kinds of honey in the United States alone, ranging in flavor from merely sweet (with little additional taste) to floral-scented. In general, lighter-colored honeys are mild in flavor, and darker honeys are more robust.

Agave Nectar: This sweetener is just hitting the shelves of some natural food stores and well-stocked grocery stores and is worth trying if you can find it. Made from a type of cactus, agave nectar comes in various grades of color and flavor. Unlike honey, agave nectar dissolves easily in cold liquids and doesn't crystallize. Ounce for ounce, agave nectar raises blood sugar less than most other natural sweeteners — that is, it has a low glycemic index.

Jams: Look for all-fruit preserves.

Extracts and Spices: Sometimes just a drop or two of vanilla or almond extract can trick your palate into thinking it is tasting sugar. Cinnamon, nutmeg, cardamom, and other "warm" spices also can give a sweet flavor without adding sugar.

Note: If you substitute liquid sweeteners such as maple syrup, honey, or agave nectar for granulated sugar in your favorite recipes, you may need to reduce other liquids to compensate for the amount of sweetener you use.

❖ Zucchini-Walnut Muffins

Yield: 8 muffins

This recipe is the ultimate in stealth nutrition. Your family will get a serving of whole grains and vegetables and probably not even know it. These muffins taste best served slightly warm the same day they are made, but they can be split in half and toasted the next day. Top with almond or peanut butter for an extra-special treat. Use an ice cream scoop with a quick-release lever to make more uniform muffins with nice rounded tops. If you are making fewer muffins than your muffin tin will hold, fill the empty muffin cups with water to promote more even baking.

1   cup whole wheat flour
2   teaspoons baking powder
1   teaspoon ground cinnamon or pumpkin pie spice
¼   teaspoon baking soda
¼   teaspoon salt
2   large egg whites
¼   cup high-oleic safflower oil, canola oil, or extra virgin olive oil
¼   cup pure maple syrup or agave nectar (see page 223)
1   teaspoon vanilla extract
1½ cups grated zucchini (about two 6-inch-long zucchini)
½   cup chopped lightly toasted walnuts (see page 211)

Preheat the oven to 350 degrees F. Lightly spray 8 muffin cups (⅓- to ½-cup capacity) with vegetable cooking spray; set aside.

In a medium bowl, combine the whole wheat flour, baking powder, cinnamon, baking soda, and salt. Whisk well to combine; set aside.

In a large mixing bowl, combine the egg whites, safflower oil, maple syrup, and vanilla extract. Using a whisk, beat the mixture vigorously until very well combined, about 1 minute. Add the zucchini and walnuts and stir until combined. Add the flour mixture all at once and stir until just combined.

Fill each muffin cup with a scant ⅓ cup batter. The batter should come nearly to the top of the cup. Fill the empty muffin cups half full of water. Bake until the tops are golden and feel firm to the touch and a wooden skewer inserted into the center of a muffin comes out clean, 20 to 25 minutes. Let the muffins cool for 10 minutes in the tin, then transfer to a wire rack.

Serve slightly warm or at room temperature. If you try to eat them while they are still hot, they will fall apart.

❖ Silky Berry-Bursting Smoothie

Yield: Two 1-cup servings

Silken tofu's extremely smooth, custardy texture makes the smoothest smoothie. For the thickest smoothie, freeze the banana and berries ahead of time. You can freeze several individual portions and just pull them out of the freezer when you want to make a smoothie. No frozen fruit? Add a few ice cubes before you puree the smoothie, or just pour over ice to serve. If you like a fruitier taste, use lemon or lime juice. If you prefer a creamier, sweeter sensation, use vanilla extract.

    1 cup mixed berries (fresh or frozen)
    1 small ripe banana, cut into thick slices (fresh or frozen)
    ⅔ cup soft silken tofu, soft regular tofu, or plain low-fat yogurt
    ¼ cup cold water or freshly squeezed orange juice
    2 teaspoons smooth peanut butter
    1 teaspoon pure maple syrup or honey (optional)
    1 teaspoon freshly squeezed lemon or lime juice or ¼ teaspoon
       vanilla extract

In a blender, combine the berries, banana, tofu, cold water, peanut butter, maple syrup (if using), and lemon juice. Puree until very smooth. Serve very cold.

GOOD FATS AND OILS

❖ Fats and oils are necessary components of a healthy diet. They provide the building blocks for cell membranes and help us absorb certain vitamins from the foods we eat. They also carry flavor in foods and help keep us full longer. But not all fats and oils are the same. We recommend the following for health, taste, and ease of use.

Extra Virgin Olive Oil: Made from the first pressing without using chemicals, extra virgin olive oil is less processed, more nutritious, and more flavorful than most other oils. It has a long shelf life and can be used in high-heat cooking or as an uncooked ingredient. Extra virgin olive oil costs more than most oils, but considering the small amount needed in recipes and the flavor it adds, it is worth the expense.

High-Oleic Safflower Oil: This relatively flavorless, odorless vegetable oil is rich in vitamin E. Make sure the label says "high-oleic," not just "safflower oil." It is the high oleic acid content that allows this oil to stand up to high-heat cooking without breaking down into unhealthy byproducts. Like extra virgin olive oil, high-oleic safflower oil has a long shelf life and can be used in high-heat cooking or as an uncooked ingredient.

Canola Oil: An all-purpose cooking oil (previously called rapeseed oil) that originated in Canada and therefore became known as Canadian or canola oil. The omega-3s in this oil can break down into unhealthy byproducts in high-heat cooking.

Butter: Because it is high in saturated fats and cholesterol, butter is not the best choice for regular use, although it is much better than partially hydrogenated (trans) fats. In addition, half a teaspoon of melted butter drizzled over steamed broccoli might make the difference between your kids eating their veggies and not eating them. Buy unsalted butter, as salt masks butter's delicate flavor. If you are cooking with butter, try a combination of half butter and half olive oil.

Store your oils in a cool, dark place and buy organic if you can.

A SIMPLE HERB, SPICE,
AND EXTRACT PANTRY

❖ A small collection of readily available dried herbs and spices, as well as vanilla and almond extracts, can add a lot of interest to very simple everyday foods. Here are a few guidelines and a list of herbs, spices, and extracts to get you started.

To ensure that your herbs, spices, and extracts taste the way you expect them to, buy the smallest quantities you can. Most herbs and spices lose their potency in six months to a year. See which ones you tend to use the most before buying them in larger quantities.

Buy whole herbs and spices whenever possible. You'll get the most flavor from dried herbs and spices (including black peppercorns) if you crush, grind, or rub them between the palms of your hands just before adding them to a recipe. A coffee grinder set aside just for spice grinding will do a fine job of grinding harder spices. Or place the spices on a large cutting board and smash them with the bottom of a heavy saucepan.

Keep your herbs, spices, and extracts in a cool, dark place. Spice racks or shelves above the stove may be pretty to look at, but the heat from the stove will zap the flavor from these products. A cool cupboard is best.

Herbs, spices, and extracts typically fall into one of three categories (savory, spicy or hot, and sweet), and those in the same category can often be substituted for one another, though not always in the same amount. A pinch of cardamom, for example, will be more than enough to stand in for a heaping teaspoon of cinnamon. If you are unsure of the potency of a particular herb or spice, start with a small amount and add more to taste. If your recipe calls for 1 tablespoon of a chopped fresh herb, you can usually substitute 1 teaspoon of the dried herb.

Finally, look for premade spice blends to save money, time, and space. Italian seasoning (a blend of basil, oregano, marjoram, and other spices typically used in Italian cooking) and poultry seasoning (a blend of savory, sage, thyme, and other spices) are available in most grocery stores, as is pumpkin pie spice (a combination of cinnamon, nutmeg, mace, and cloves). Be sure to read the label on any blends to make sure you are buying a blend of herbs and spices *not* flavored with salt and MSG.

Savory	Spicy or Hot	Sweet
Basil	Black pepper	Almond extract
Bay leaves	Cayenne pepper	Cardamom
Dill weed	Chili powder	Cinnamon
Garlic powder	Cloves	Coriander
Marjoram	Cumin	Mace
Onion powder or flakes	Curry powder	Nutmeg
Oregano	Ginger	Vanilla extract
Parsley	Hot paprika	
Rosemary	Red pepper flakes	
Sage	Sweet Hungarian	
Tarragon	paprika	
Thyme		
Turmeric		

A FEW WORDS ABOUT COOKWARE

❖ Go into any kitchen store, and you will find an overwhelming variety of pots and pans. The choice is personal — color, weight, and style — but it can be helpful to know a few of the pros and cons of each material and coating.

Cookware

❖ *Cast Iron:* Cast-iron cookware is heavy and can withstand very high temperatures. Cast iron can be purchased preseasoned, or you can season it after purchase according to the manufacturer's instructions to make it nearly nonstick. To retain its seasoning, cast iron should be washed according to the manufacturer's instructions and thoroughly dried to avoid rust.

Stainless Steel: Stainless steel cookware is usually made with an insert of copper or aluminum in the base to improve its heat conductivity. These pots and pans vary in weight depending on the thickness of the steel and the type of insert used. Stainless steel itself resists corrosion, scratches, and dents. There is a trick to help prevent food from sticking to the surface of a stainless steel pan: Heat the empty pan over medium-high to high heat. When the pan is hot, add the oil. When the oil is hot, add the food and cook undisturbed. The food will naturally release from the pan as it browns.

Coatings

❖ *Enamel:* An enamel coating is often applied over cast iron to create an almost nonstick surface. Enamel-coated cookware is nonreactive to acidic foods. Enamel coatings are also applied to stainless steel cookware. Enamel can chip if dropped or knocked onto a hard surface.

Nonstick: Nonstick cookware is coated with a substance to reduce the possibility of food sticking to the pan. Because some of these coatings can break down into toxic products at high temperatures, nonstick cookware should be used only over moderate or low heat. Care should be taken to use wooden or other nonmetal utensils when stirring or scraping so as not to scratch the coating off the pan and into the food.

HOW TO READ A NUTRITION FACTS FOOD LABEL AND A LIST OF INGREDIENTS

❖ *The Nutrition Facts Label* found on all packaged foods (see Figure 9.1) contains lots of information to help you make healthy choices. Consider the following when comparing packaged foods.

Start with the *serving size,* found at the top of the label, just under the name of the product. This will tell you how big a serving is (1 cup in the sample label). Underneath is the *servings per container* (10 servings in the sample label). All the other numbers on the label are based on a single serving of the product. Therefore, if you eat twice the serving size indicated, you'll be getting twice the calories and twice of everything else on the list.

Calories are a way of measuring the energy contained in food. Fats have 9 calories per gram; carbohydrates and protein have 4 calories per gram. In the sample label, 18 calories come from fats, 160 calories from carbohydrates (not counting fiber), and 20 calories from protein, for a total of about 200 calories. Remember, the calories listed are *per serving,* not per package.

Total fat, total carbohydrate, and *protein* tell you where the calories in the food come from. For example, if a product is advertised as high protein, check to see how the number of protein grams compares with the number of fat and carbohydrate grams.

Ultimately, the most important aspect of the food we eat is its *quality.* Instead of just focusing on whether a product is low fat or low carbohydrate, look at what kinds of fats and carbohydrates are present. Choose products with lower amounts of saturated fats, and avoid any items with trans fats completely. For carbohydrate-containing foods (bread, cereals, baked goods), the more fiber, the better.

❖ *The List of Ingredients* indicates what ingredients are actually in a product, in decreasing order. That means that the first ingredient on the list makes up the largest proportion of the food. Read the list of ingredients carefully. Look to see if sugar (including sucrose, dextrose, fructose, corn syrup, or dextran) is one of the first few ingredients. Avoid foods with partially hydrogenated (trans) fats. And if a product has ingredients that you can't pronounce, think twice before buying it.

Nutrition Facts

Serving Size 1 cup (54g/1.9oz)
Servings Per Container about 10

Amount Per Serving

Calories 200	Calories from Fat 20

	% Daily Value*
Total Fat 2g	3%
Saturated Fat 0g	0%
Trans Fat 0g	
Cholesterol 0g	0%
Sodium 130mg	5%
Total Carbohydrate 45g	15%
Dietary Fiber 6g	24%
Sugars 7g	
Protein 5g	

Vitamin A 0%	•	Vitamin C 0%
Calcium 2%	•	Iron 8%

* Percent Daily Values are based on a 2,000 calorie diet. Your Daily Values may be higher or lower depending on your calorie needs.

	Calories	2,000	2,500
Total Fat	Less than	65g	80g
Sat Fat	Less than	20g	25g
Cholesterol	Less than	300mg	300mg
Sodium	Less than	2,400mg	2,400mg
Total Carbohydrate		300mg	375mg
Dietary Fiber		25g	30g

Calories per gram:
Fat 9   *   Carbohydrate 4   *   Protein 4

Figure 9.1 Sample Nutrition Label for a Whole Grain Cereal

What's for Lunch?

It's sad but true: almost anything is better than today's cafeteria school lunch. Even if a school wants to implement a healthy lunch program, a lack of financial support and the maze of government regulations (sometimes protecting corporate interests over the health of our children) can become nearly insurmountable obstacles.

But you don't have to take it. Well, actually, you *do* have to take it — your lunch that is. Pack up a delicious and nutritious meal so that your child can skip standing in the long cafeteria line to obesity and other health problems. Making a healthy, tasty lunch can be a quick, even enjoyable routine if you get yourself set up with the right equipment and ingredients.

To start, your child will need some way to carry his lunch to school. Keep in mind that peer pressure is real — and if it's not cool, it's not going to school. Your job as a parent is to use that peer pressure to your advantage. So get your child involved in picking out an insulated lunch bag, a lunch box, or even simple brown paper bags. If you make taking lunch to school a cool thing, you just might find you've started a trend among your kid's friends.

If you are going to make lunch every day, you'll want to be organized in the kitchen and familiar with the basics of sandwich making. With very little effort and time, you can set up a small area of your kitchen to make preparing lunches a snap. See Pack It Up! (page 223) for some specific items that will come in handy every day. To familiarize yourself with the basics of a tasty, healthy sandwich, check out Sandwich 101 (page 234).

Food safety is important but not difficult to maintain. Keep cold foods cold and hot foods hot. If you pack an item that you would normally keep in the refrigerator at home, use an ice pack in the lunch bag. Hot foods should travel in a thermos or vacuum flask. To keep foods as hot as possible, rinse the thermos with boiling water just before filling, heat the food as hot as possible before you put it in the thermos, and fill the thermos as close to capacity as you can. Fortunately, most lunch bag favorites can be kept at room temperature if your child is going to have lunch within four to six hours.

Remember, lunch is not the time to aim for dietary perfection or culinary masterpieces. It is the time to provide your child with a healthier alternative to the cafeteria lunch and to make it one he will actually eat. The no-muss, no-fuss Mix-and-Match Sandwich Table (page 236) will allow you to make a nearly limitless variety of sandwiches. If your child feels like a change from sandwiches, the other recipes in this section won't take a lot of work or extra time to make. Don't miss the "Lunch Bag Tips" at the end of each recipe in this section.

PACK IT UP!

❖ Packing a lunch in the wee hours of the morning will be easy and fast if you set aside a drawer, a small cupboard, or even a portion of the countertop to store your child's lunch bag and thermos, along with a small collection of plastic or other travel-safe bowls, containers, and utensils. Keeping these items close at hand will eliminate the need to rummage around the kitchen when you really need to be getting out the door and on your way. Here are some of the most useful items to have on hand.

- Square, sandwich-size containers with tight-fitting lids to keep sandwiches looking and tasting their best. They are also the perfect size to carry leftovers from dinner.
- Two-cup bowls with tight-fitting lids (or similar-capacity shallow, rectangular containers) to transport salads and such. You want to have a little extra room so your child can toss the salad with the dressing at lunchtime.

- One-quarter- to ½-cup containers with tight-fitting lids to fill with dips, salad dressings, and other toppings.
- Plastic wrap, wax paper, aluminum foil, and resealable plastic sandwich bags.
- A 10-ounce, wide-mouth thermos or vacuum flask to keep hot foods hot. Look for one with a lid that doubles as a serving bowl. Some even come with a built-in spoon holder.
- Ice packs to keep cold foods cold. These come in two versions: hard-sided (durable, but take up a bit more room) and soft-sided (less durable, but thinner). It's useful to have at least two — one can be in use while the other is being washed and frozen.
- Plastic forks, spoons, and knives.
- Napkins.

All of these items can be found in a well-stocked grocery store. As you fall into a lunch-making routine, you might want containers of other sizes and shapes to fit your child's own eating style. Try looking in an Asian grocery or hardware store for a source of small, cool-looking plastic and metal containers with tight-fitting lids. If you have trouble finding containers small enough to hold just a tablespoon or two of salad dressing, look in the spice or international food aisle of your grocery store. Many of the products found there come in plastic bottles and jars that are just the right size for this purpose (once you've used their original contents). There are even online sources of containers. Be creative — but make sure that all containers are made of food-safe plastic or another unbreakable material and that they are appropriate for your child's age.

SANDWICH 101

❖ *Merriam-Webster's Collegiate Dictionary* defines a sandwich as "two or more slices of bread with a filling . . . in between." Quite doable — even at 6:00 A.M. and before your first cup of coffee. Assembling a great sandwich is not rocket science, and just a few tips will make you an expert.

Bread

❖ There may be an entire aisle of bread in the grocery store. How on earth will you ever be able to find a healthy, good-tasting one? Read the labels. Whether you've chosen wheat, rye, barley, rice, buckwheat, millet, or spelt bread, make sure the first word in the list of ingredients is "whole." It's even better if it says "stone-ground." And you've hit the nutritional jackpot if it says "whole kernel," "wheat berry," "sprouted," or "flourless." Don't be tricked by "wheat flour," "unbleached wheat flour," or "enriched wheat flour." If it doesn't say "whole," the bran and germ (and their accompanying nutrients and fiber) have been refined out, and a little molasses, brown sugar, or even artificial color has been put in to give it that whole wheat bread color. Also look for a bread with at least 3 grams of fiber per serving.

And don't be afraid to think outside the breadbox. Your whole grain can come in the form of whole grain tortillas, whole grain English muffins, or even whole grain crackers.

Spreads and Dressings

❖ Most sandwiches benefit from at least a little spread or dressing on the bread or in the filling. Mustard, ketchup, and mayonnaise are the obvious choices. A one-tablespoon serving of mayonnaise is usually more than sufficient for an entire sandwich. Replace the mayonnaise with creamy, garlicky hummus in a fresh or grilled vegetable sandwich for more intense flavor and zing. Use guacamole instead of mayonnaise with chicken, cheese, or vegetables. You might skip the spread altogether if you drizzle the sandwich filling with a little Basic Vinaigrette (page 274) or extra virgin olive oil.

Filling Textures and Flavors

❖ Texture is an important consideration when making a sandwich. If all the ingredients are soft and squishy, the sandwich will be somewhat boring. But if you make an effort to vary the textures a bit — say by adding some crunchy lettuce, thin slices of cucumber, or chopped red pepper — your sandwich will take on a whole new personality. Lettuce or spinach can be left as is, torn into bite-size pieces, or cut into thin ribbons that are more easily stuffed into a pita. Each will give a different texture to your sandwich.

Finally, don't shortchange the taste buds. A flavorful sandwich will make your child want to take her lunch to school every day. Beyond the flavor of the bread, the spread, and the filling, you can add even more zip with salt and pepper or a sprinkling of fresh or dried herbs.

❖ "Your Name Here" Specialty Sandwich

Yield: 1 sandwich

If you are unsure of what to put on your child's sandwich, or if you find yourself stuck in a rut when it comes to making lunch, use the following table. Pick an item from each column to create your very own specialty sandwich.

THE MIX-AND-MATCH SANDWICH TABLE

Select an item from each column — you can choose two or more from the vegetables and the herbs and seasonings columns — and assemble as a sandwich.

Bread	Protein	Vegetables	Spreads and Dressings	Herbs and Seasonings
Multigrain bread (2 slices)	Cheese (2 ounces)	Baby spinach	Extra virgin olive oil	Balsamic or red wine vinegar
		Bell peppers		
		Cucumbers	Guacamole	

Bread	Protein	Vegetables	Spreads and Dressings	Herbs and Seasonings
Whole grain English muffins (1 whole muffin)	Chicken (3 ounces)	Lettuce	Hummus	Dried herbs: basil, dill, tarragon, thyme, oregano,
	Egg salad (1/4 cup)	Mushrooms	Ketchup	Italian seasoning,
Whole grain pita bread (1 whole pita)		Onions	Mayonnaise	or other premixed herb or spice blend
	Salmon (3 ounces)	Pepperoncini (deli-style pickled hot peppers)	Mustard	
Whole brain pumpernickel bread (2 slices)	Tuna salad (1/4 cup)		Relish	Fresh herbs: parsley, cilantro, basil
		Pickles	Salsa	Salt and pepper
Whole grain rye bread (2 slices)	Turkey (3 ounces)	Raw, grilled, steamed,		
	Vegetarian cold cuts (4 ounces)	sautéed, or blanched vegetables (see page 257)		
Whole grain tortillas (one 7-inch tortilla)				
Whole grain wheat bread (2 slices)		Sprouts		
		Tomatoes		

Lunch Bag Tips

WRAP the sandwich tightly in aluminum foil, wax paper, or plastic wrap, or use a resealable plastic sandwich bag.

STORE in an insulated lunch bag, brown bag, or lunch box. KEEP cool.

SERVE with carrot and celery sticks packed separately in a small resealable plastic bag or travel-safe container.

QUICK PICK!

❖ ANB&J (Any Nut Butter and Jam) Sandwich

Yield: 1 sandwich

There will be days when all you have time to do is spread some peanut butter on one slice of bread, spread some jam on another, and slap the two together. Add an apple, and you're good to go. Luckily, in addition to being quick and easy, it's also tasty and nutritious. And if you tire of peanut butter, try any nut butter (almond, cashew, pecan, hazelnut, macadamia).

Most natural food stores and many grocery stores stock nut butters right next to the peanut butter. Skip over any that include sugar and partially hydrogenated (trans) fats. The only ingredients listed on the nut butter jar should be nuts and salt. As for jams and jellies, you might be surprised how many are mostly sugar with a little fruit added for flavor. The first ingredient listed on the jar should be fruit, and the farther down the list you find any type of sugar, the better. You can also substitute thinly sliced banana or other soft fruit for the jam.

- 2 tablespoons nut butter
- 2 slices whole grain bread
- 2–3 teaspoons fruit jam or ½ banana, thinly sliced

Spread the nut butter on one slice of bread and the jam on the other. Place them together, and you're done. (Alternatively, put a thin layer of nut butter on both slices before topping with the jam. The nut butter will keep the jam from soaking into the bread.)

Lunch Bag Tips

WRAP the sandwich tightly in aluminum foil, wax paper, or plastic wrap, or use a resealable plastic sandwich bag.

STORE in an insulated lunch bag, brown bag, or lunch box.
KEEP at room temperature.
SERVE with a crisp fresh apple.

❖ Pita Pizza

Yield: 2 sandwiches

Fast food restaurants mass-produce it, convenience stores sell it micro-wavable, and schools defrost it, but you can make pizza healthy and portable. For a really fresh flavor, try making your own pizza sauce. If you use store-bought pizza or spaghetti sauce, check the label to make sure sugar is not one of the first three ingredients.

One 7-inch whole grain pita bread
3–4 tablespoons Basic Pasta and Pizza Sauce (page 280) or
     store-bought pizza or spaghetti sauce
¼ cup crumbled ready-to-eat veggie sausage
2 tablespoons shredded mozzarella or Monterey Jack cheese
2 teaspoons chopped fresh basil or big pinch of dried basil
2 teaspoons freshly grated Parmesan cheese
Mixed lettuce (such as red leaf, green leaf, and romaine),
     coarsely chopped

Cut the pita bread in half and gently open both pockets. Spread the inside of each pita pocket with 1½ to 2 tablespoons of the sauce. Scatter 2 tablespoons of the veggie sausage, 1 tablespoon of the mozzarella, 1 teaspoon of the basil, and 1 teaspoon of the Parmesan evenly over the pizza sauce in each pita pocket. Fill any leftover space with chopped lettuce.

Lunch Bag Tips

WRAP the pita tightly in aluminum foil, wax paper, or plastic
wrap.

STORE in an insulated lunch bag, brown bag, or lunch box.

KEEP cool.

SERVE with a handful of cherry tomatoes packed separately
in a small resealable plastic bag or travel-safe container.

PUT MORE GREEN IN YOUR LUNCH BAG

❖ You can lessen your impact on the earth by packing a "greener"
lunch that reduces the amount of trash you create. Save money and
save the planet.

Pack sandwiches in reusable travel-safe containers instead of
using aluminum foil, wax paper, or plastic wrap that will be thrown
away. Pack drinks in reusable, unbreakable bottles instead of buying them in boxes. And pack everything in an insulated lunch bag
or box instead of a disposable bag.

Use cloth napkins. Include two — one to use as a place mat
for lunch and to clean up messes and spills and one for wiping
hands and face.

Look for biodegradable forks, spoons, and knives. If you can't
find these eco-friendly utensils, just wash and reuse your plastic
utensils.

❖ BBQ Chicken Roll-Up

Yield: 1 large sandwich or 2 small sandwiches

Your child will enjoy the flavor of a summer barbecue rolled up in her lunch box. The dressing combines mayonnaise and yogurt for a tangy salad that pairs perfectly with the smoky taste of the chicken filling. When choosing barbecue sauce, look for a brand with as little sugar as possible.

Salad
1 tablespoon plain low-fat yogurt
1 tablespoon mayonnaise
1 tablespoon chopped green onions
1 cup finely shredded white, green, or red cabbage
Salt and freshly ground black pepper

Filling
3 ounces cooked chicken, shredded, or 4 ounces savory baked
   tofu, cut into matchsticks
1½–2 tablespoons store-bought barbecue sauce
Salt and freshly ground black pepper

One 9-inch or two 7-inch whole grain tortillas

To make the salad: In a medium bowl, whisk together the yogurt, mayonnaise, and green onions until well combined. Add the cabbage and toss to coat evenly. Season with salt and pepper to taste.

To make the filling: In a small bowl, combine the chicken and barbecue sauce. Toss well to coat. Season with salt and pepper to taste.

To assemble the sandwich(es): If making 1 large sandwich, spread the filling down the center of the 9-inch tortilla, stopping about 2 inches from the bottom edge. Top with the salad and roll up burrito-style. If making 2 small sandwiches, divide the filling and salad evenly between two 7-inch tortillas and roll up.

Lunch Bag Tips

> WRAP the roll-up tightly in aluminum foil, wax paper, or
> plastic wrap.
> STORE in an insulated lunch bag, brown bag, or lunch box.
> KEEP cool.
> SERVE with a juicy orange.

❖ Fake'n, Lettuce, and Tomato Sandwich

Yield: 1 sandwich

This is the sandwich to celebrate summer, and it's worth waiting for. Start with the reddest, ripest tomato you can find. Add crisp lettuce and savory vegetarian bacon strips. Then sit down and enjoy. This sandwich doesn't travel well, so make it at home on a lazy summer afternoon.

1 tablespoon mayonnaise
2 slices hearty whole grain bread, lightly toasted
3 or 4 small fresh basil leaves, whole or chopped
2 or 3 red leaf or romaine lettuce leaves
2 slices (about 2 ounces) mozzarella or Monterey Jack cheese
2 or 3 veggie bacon strips, cooked
2 or 3 large slices ripe tomato
Salt and freshly ground black pepper

Spread ½ tablespoon of the mayonnaise evenly on one slice of toast. Top with the basil leaves, lettuce, cheese, veggie bacon strips, and tomato. Season with salt and pepper to taste. Spread the remaining ½ tablespoon mayonnaise on the other slice of toast and place on top of the tomato. Serve immediately.

Lunch Bag Tips

If you absolutely must take this sandwich with you, don't toast the bread and pack the tomato separately.

> WRAP the sandwich tightly in aluminum foil, wax paper, or plastic wrap, or use a resealable plastic sandwich bag. Wrap the tomato slices separately in plastic wrap or place in a small travel-safe container.
> STORE in an insulated lunch bag, brown bag, or lunch box.
> KEEP cool.
> SERVE by adding the tomato slices to the sandwich when you are ready to eat it. Accompany with a small bag of chips — just make sure there are no partially hydrogenated (trans) fats in them.

❖ Tuna Salad

Yield: 2 servings

Tuna salad doesn't have to be laden with mayonnaise to be tasty. Here the mayonnaise and pickle juice add just the right amount of creaminess to the salad. Like all recipes with few ingredients, the quality of those ingredients really counts. For this recipe, look for dolphin-safe tuna packed in spring water and hearty whole grain crackers. Canned salmon or firm tofu is a nice alternative to tuna.

1 tablespoon mayonnaise
1 teaspoon yellow mustard
2 teaspoons finely chopped dill pickle plus 1 tablespoon dill pickle juice

2 teaspoons finely minced yellow onion
One 6-ounce can water-packed tuna, drained; one 6-ounce can
   salmon, drained; or 1 cup diced firm regular tofu
Salt and freshly ground black pepper
Whole grain crackers

In a small bowl, combine the mayonnaise, mustard, pickle and pickle juice, and onion. Mix well. Add the tuna and mix until well combined. Season with salt and pepper to taste. Serve with whole grain crackers.

Lunch Bag Tips

WRAP the crackers in plastic wrap or place in a small travel-
   safe container. Pack half of the tuna mixture in a small
   travel-safe container with a tight-fitting lid. (The remaining
   tuna mixture will keep, refrigerated, for up to 2 days.)
STORE in an insulated lunch bag, brown bag, or lunch box
   and include a fork.
KEEP cold with a frozen ice pack.
SERVE with a slice of melon.

❖ Greek Salad

Yield: 2 servings

Use Roma, or plum, tomatoes in this recipe, if you can. Romas have fewer seeds and thicker flesh than other kinds of tomatoes, so they don't squish as easily when tossed with the other ingredients. If you don't like to peel cucumbers, look for the long, skinny English cucumbers, which have mild-tasting skins that can be left on when slicing and dicing for salads. Of course, you can use any olives you like, but the purple-black Kalamata olives will give your salad an authentic Greek taste. You'll find hummus, the classic Middle Eastern spread made from chickpeas, in the refrigerator section of your grocery store, near the fresh dips and salsas.

1 cup cored and diced Roma tomatoes
1 cup peeled and diced cucumber
½ cup chopped red bell pepper
12 pitted Kalamata olives, whole or coarsely chopped
2 tablespoons chopped red onion
1 tablespoon freshly squeezed lemon juice
2 teaspoons extra virgin olive oil
¼–½ teaspoon finely minced garlic (optional)
¼ teaspoon chopped fresh oregano or big pinch of dried oregano
Salt and freshly ground black pepper
½ cup crumbled feta cheese (optional)

Whole grain crackers, for serving
Store-bought hummus, for serving

In a small bowl, combine the tomatoes, cucumber, bell pepper, olives, onion, lemon juice, olive oil, garlic (if using), and oregano. Toss to combine. Season with salt and pepper to taste.

Divide the salad evenly between two plates and top with the feta, if using. Serve with whole grain crackers and hummus on the side.

Lunch Bag Tips

WRAP the crackers in plastic wrap or place in a small travel-safe container. Place half of the salad in a 2-cup travel-safe bowl with a tight-fitting lid. (The remaining salad will keep, refrigerated, for up to 1 day.) Top with half of the feta, if using. Place the hummus in a small travel-safe container with a tight-fitting lid.

STORE in an insulated lunch bag, brown bag, or lunch box and include a fork and knife.

KEEP cool.

SERVE with the crackers and hummus on the side.

QUICK PICK!

❖ Soup's On!

Sandwiches and salads make great lunches, but on a cold winter day, nothing warms you up like a bowl of hot soup. Add a wedge of cheese and some whole grain crackers on the side, and you have a complete meal.

The choice of soups in most grocery stores is almost overwhelming. Besides canned soups, many stores now carry frozen or refrigerated soups. Not all soups are created equal, so choose carefully. The list of ingredients ought to include foods you recognize, not a lot of chemicals. Also keep an eye out for high sodium levels. Stick to vegetable and bean combinations for the healthiest soups. Black bean soup or chili, vegetarian chili, and minestrone are some of the more kid-friendly flavors.

1 can of soup
One 2-ounce cheese wedge
Whole grain crackers

Open the can of soup and heat according to the package directions. You may or may not need to add water — the instructions on the label will tell you.

Transfer the soup to a serving bowl. (The number of servings per can or container will vary, so read the label for guidance.)

Serve with the cheese and a handful of whole grain crackers on the side.

Lunch Bag Tips

WRAP the cheese and crackers separately in plastic wrap or place in small travel-safe containers. Pour a serving of hot soup into a preheated thermos or vacuum flask and close tightly.

STORE in an insulated lunch bag, brown bag, or lunch box and include a spoon.

KEEP the cheese cool — not in direct contact with the hot thermos.

SERVE with the cheese and crackers on the side.

❖ Kabobs — Red, White, and Green

Yield: 1 serving

Cubes of mozzarella cheese, cherry tomatoes, and broccoli florets line up on skewers, ready to get a dunking in a basil-flavored yogurt dip. This is a fun way to get kids to eat healthily — and the kabobs make great party food, too. If you want to make enough for several days' lunches at once, refrigerate the mozzarella, tomatoes, and blanched broccoli in separate containers and skewer just what you need for lunch that day. The yogurt dip can be made in a larger batch and will keep, refrigerated, for 3 to 4 days.

Four 1-inch cubes mozzarella
4 cherry tomatoes
4 bite-size broccoli florets, blanched (see page 258)

¼ cup plain low-fat yogurt
1 tablespoon finely chopped fresh basil

¼ teaspoon finely minced garlic
Salt and freshly ground black pepper

Arrange the cheese, tomatoes, and broccoli florets in pleasing patterns on two to four 6- to 8-inch wooden skewers. (*Note:* If serving to young children, skip the skewers and serve the cheese, tomatoes, and broccoli in a bowl.) In a small bowl, combine the yogurt, basil, and garlic. Season with salt and pepper to taste. To eat, dip the kabob, bite by bite, into the yogurt mixture.

Lunch Bag Tips

WRAP the kabobs tightly in plastic wrap or place in a travel-safe container. Place the dip in a small travel-safe bowl with a tight-fitting lid.
STORE in an insulated lunch bag, brown bag, or lunch box.
KEEP cool.
SERVE with a handful of nuts.

QUICK PICK!

❖ Fruit and Cheese with Crackers

Yield: 1 serving

This "recipe" proves that there is really no excuse for not making your child a lunch. You overslept? No problem — this takes just a minute to assemble. And if the refrigerator is empty and the cupboard bare, it's still not a problem. You can pull this together with a quick dash into almost any mini-mart along your way. It doesn't get any easier than this.

1 apple
2 slices deli-style cheese, 2 individually wrapped cheese sticks, or two 1-inch cheese cubes
Whole grain crackers

Enjoy!

Lunch Bag Tips

WRAP the cheese and crackers separately in plastic wrap or place in small travel-safe containers.

STORE in an insulated lunch bag, brown bag, or lunch box.

KEEP cool.

SERVE the apple, cheese, and crackers together.

Dinner Is Served

With a busy family going in who knows how many different directions, there are days when the thought of having to come up with an idea for dinner is enough to drive you crazy — or at least to the nearest takeout restaurant. Just this once, you tell yourself, and before you know it, dinner becomes a fast food affair.

But you don't have to go down that road. For a simple, no-nonsense approach to dinner, use The Basic Meal section to design a balanced meal. Choose a protein, vegetable, salad, and whole grain from the Mix-and-Match Basic Meal Planner (page 251), follow the cooking instructions in the foolproof guides (pages 252–266), and then use the Portion Proportions (page 265) and the Guide to Serving Size (page 301) to determine serving sizes.

For those nights you have a little more time, try one of the recipes in Putting It All Together. Spaghetti Veggie Medley (page 266), Salad Bar Stir-Fry with Tofu or Chicken (page 268), Fajitas (page 275), and Pizza Anytime (page 277) are all great options that kids and adults will love. Either way, you can have a healthful, filling, and tasty meal on the table every night without spending all day in the kitchen.

The Basic Meal

Mix-and-Match Basic Meal Planner

It takes almost no effort to figure out the components of a healthy, balanced dinner using the Mix-and-Match Basic Meal Planner. Pick an item from each column of the table, and voilà! — you have your dinner plan. Don't worry about menu fatigue and boredom; the items in the columns can be combined in nearly endless combinations.

MIX-AND-MATCH BASIC MEAL PLANNER

Select one item from each columns. For suggestions on cooking protein, vegetables, salads, whole grains, and potatoes, see the foolproof guides on pages 252–266. For a guide to portion size, see page 265.

Protein	Vegetables	Salad: Choose one or a combination of items.	Whole Grains and Potatoes
Beans	Asparagus	Cabbage	Amaranth
Chicken	Beets	Carrots	Brown rice
Eggs	Bell peppers	Cucumbers	Hulled barley
Fish	Broccoli	Lettuce:	Millet
Seitan	Cabbage	romaine, butter,	Pearl barley
Soy: tofu and tempeh	Carrots	green leaf, red	Quinoa
	Cauliflower	leaf, iceberg	Wheat berries
	Chard	Radishes	Wild rice
	Collard greens	Spinach	
	Eggplant	Tomatoes	Potatoes
	Green beans or		Sweet potatoes
	wax beans		Yams
	Kale		
	Mustard greens		
	Onions		
	Parsnips		
	Peas		
	Rutabagas		
	Spinach		
	Summer squash		
	Tomatoes		
	Turnips		
	Winter squash		

The Foolproof Guide to Cooking Protein

Cooking chicken, fish, tofu, tempeh, eggs, and beans doesn't have to be intimidating, even if you're not an accomplished cook. Check out the following suggestions for tips on how to get some tasty, simply cooked protein on your dinner plate with the minimum amount of time and effort. Of course, there are many other ways to prepare protein. You can poach fish, broil chicken, and cook beans in a soup, for example. There are hundreds of cookbooks to show you how, but the following quick, easy, and reliable recipes will get you on your way in a hurry.

CHICKEN

Sautéed Boneless Chicken Breasts, With or Without Skin

3 ounces equals 1 serving

Season 6- to 8-ounce boneless chicken breasts, with or without the skin, with salt, pepper, and your favorite herb(s) (thyme, rosemary, sage, and savory all go well with chicken). Set aside. Heat a skillet over medium-high heat until hot. Add a tablespoon or so of extra virgin olive oil and swirl to coat the bottom of the pan. Add the chicken breasts (skin side down, if still attached) and cook, undisturbed, until browned on the bottom, 5 to 7 minutes for smaller breasts and 7 to 9 minutes for larger ones. (You may need to turn the heat up or down just a bit depending on your pan and stove. You want the skillet hot enough for the chicken to brown and cook quickly, but not so hot that the chicken burns before it's cooked through.) Turn the breasts over and continue to cook until golden brown on the other side and no longer pink inside, 5 to 7 minutes more for smaller breasts and 7 to 9 minutes more for larger ones. Transfer the breasts to a plate and let rest for 2 to 3 minutes before serving.

Baked Chicken Legs and Thighs, With or Without Skin

1 leg or thigh (5–6 ounces) equals 1 serving

Preheat the oven to 425 degrees F. Lightly oil a roasting pan or baking dish. If the legs and/or thighs are skinless, brush lightly with extra virgin olive oil. Season generously with salt, pepper, and your favorite herb(s) (thyme, rosemary, sage, and savory all go well with chicken). Place (skin side up, if still attached) in the prepared pan. Bake, undisturbed, until golden brown and the juices run clear when the chicken is pierced with a fork, about 45 minutes. Transfer to a plate and let rest for 5 minutes before serving.

If you have time, you can marinate legs and thighs before baking. After you season the chicken, toss the pieces into a resealable plastic bag. Add a few tablespoons of extra virgin olive oil (you want just enough oil to coat all the chicken evenly) and a teaspoon or two of minced garlic. Seal the bag and squish it around to coat the chicken with the oil and garlic. Refrigerate for at least 30 minutes or up to overnight. When ready to cook, remove the chicken from the bag, pat dry with paper towels, and cook as described.

FISH

Oven-Broiled Fish Fillets, With or Without Skin

3 ounces equals 1 serving

Adjust the oven rack so that your fish fillets will be 4 to 5 inches below the broiler's heat source. Preheat the broiler and broiler pan (or a broiler-safe baking sheet). Brush 1-inch-thick fish fillets with extra virgin olive oil and season generously with salt and pepper. Place (skin side down, if still attached) on the preheated pan. Broil for 4 to 5 minutes. Carefully turn the fillets over and broil for 4 to 5 minutes more. When done, the fish will be opaque and flake easily when nudged with a fork. (As a rule, you need to cook fish 8 to 10 minutes total for every inch of thickness.) Take care not to overcook, or it will be dry. Serve with a lemon or lime wedge.

SOY

Pan-Fried Tofu and Tempeh

4 ounces equals 1 serving

One trick to producing a browned and slightly crisp piece of pan-fried tofu (see page 216) or tempeh (see page 256) is to use the proper spatula for turning the slices. A thin, flexible spatula — the type you would use to flip pancakes or fried eggs — works best. A thin spatula will slide easily between the crust that forms on the surface of the tofu or tempeh and the pan. A thicker spatula tends to scrape off the crust and leave it sticking to the pan. It is not a culinary disaster if this happens, but the crust adds a nice texture and flavor.

Slice firm or extra-firm regular tofu, baked tofu, or tempeh into ½-inch-thick slabs. Heat a skillet over medium heat until hot. Add a tablespoon or so of extra virgin olive oil or high-oleic safflower oil and swirl to generously coat the bottom of the pan. Add the tofu or tempeh in a single layer and cook, undisturbed, until browned on the bottom, 5 to 10 minutes. Turn the slices over and cook for another 5 to 10 minutes. Season with soy sauce or teriyaki sauce to taste.

EGGS

Soft- or Hard-Boiled

1 egg equals 1 serving

Select a saucepan that will hold the eggs in a single layer (with just a bit of wiggle room) and enough water to cover them by about 1 inch. Prepare a bowl of ice water to plunge the eggs into as soon as they come off the stove.

Bring the water to a boil (without the eggs) over high heat. Using a spoon, carefully lower the eggs into the water. When the water returns to a boil, reduce the heat to low and cook at a simmer for 3 to 4 minutes for soft-boiled or 10 minutes for hard-boiled. Immediately drain the eggs and transfer to the ice water to stop the cooking and make peeling easier.

BEANS

½ cup equals 1 serving as a side dish; 1 cup equals 1 serving as a main dish

Although you can cook beans from scratch, canned versions are usually more convenient. Whether you are planning to use the canned beans cold, at room temperature, or reheated, rinse them thoroughly under cold running water and drain them well. This will wash away most of the indigestible sugars that can cause intestinal gas. To reheat canned beans, place the beans in a saucepan with 1 to 2 tablespoons water for every 15-ounce can of beans. Cover and cook over medium heat, stirring often, until hot. If any water remains, drain the beans and discard the liquid. Season with salt and pepper to taste. If you plan to serve the beans on their own, you might want to drizzle them with

---

MEAT SUBSTITUTES: TEMPEH AND SEITAN

❖ *Tempeh* is a versatile, protein-rich meat substitute made from soybeans that have been cooked and then fermented. The resulting firm, chewy cake has a savory, nutty flavor. You'll find tempeh next to tofu in the refrigerator section of natural food stores, Asian markets, and some grocery stores. It should be used within 1 week of opening the package. It can be frozen for up to 6 months. Pure soybean tempeh can be a bit bitter. If you like a mellower taste, look for tempeh containing rye, millet, rice, or other grains. Tempeh can be added as is to soups and stews or pan- or stir-fried to give it a crunchy crust.

Seitan is another high-protein meat substitute. It is sometimes sold as *wheat gluten, wheat meat,* or *wheat roast.* Seitan chunks or cutlets packaged in a light broth or flavored marinade are found next to tofu in the refrigerator section of natural food stores and some grocery stores. It also might be found in the freezer section or with the canned goods (in jars of broth). Seitan should be used within 1 week of opening the container. It can be frozen for about 6 months. Seitan can get tough if overcooked, so it's best to cook it in hot oil just long enough to brown or to heat it through in broth or sauce.

---

extra virgin olive oil and add a pinch of dried or fresh herbs. Basil, tarragon, and thyme all complement white beans nicely. Oregano, marjoram, Italian seasoning, and ground cumin go well with red beans, pinto beans, and black beans. Grated cheese and salsa make nice toppings.

The Foolproof Guide to Cooking Vegetables

Cooking vegetables is simple. Pick a vegetable, pick a cooking method, consult the table on page 259 for estimated cooking time, and go.

Plan on making at least 1 cup of vegetables per person. Extra virgin olive oil, salt, and freshly ground black pepper are all you need for seasoning.

Sautéing

Heat a skillet over medium-high heat. (Make sure the skillet is large enough to give the vegetables room to move. If they are crowded, they will steam rather than sauté.) Add enough extra virgin olive oil to coat the bottom of the skillet. When the oil is hot, add the vegetables and cook, stirring frequently, until tender. Season with salt and pepper to taste and serve.

Some sturdy greens such as chard, collards, and kale cook best if you wilt them a bit before sautéing. Add 2 to 3 tablespoons water to the pan after you add the greens. Immediately cover the pan and let the greens wilt for 2 to 3 minutes. Remove the lid and continue to cook until tender. Any excess water will evaporate once the lid is removed.

Steaming

Steaming will require a steamer insert or a collapsible steamer basket (a perforated metal "bowl" with petal-like sides that flare in or out to adjust to the size of your pot).

Bring approximately 2 inches of water to a boil in the bottom of a steamer or saucepan fitted with a steamer basket. The boiling water should not touch the bottom of the insert or basket. Add the vegetables, cover tightly, and cook until tender. Season with salt and pepper to taste and serve.

Boiling

Place 1 cup water for every 1 cup vegetable you plan to cook in a saucepan and bring to a boil over high heat. Lightly salt the water and add the vegetables. Cook until tender. Drain well, season with salt and pepper to taste, and serve.

Blanching

Blanching is the perfect method for cooking vegetables you want to use in a tossed salad or as crudités. It takes away the rawness but leaves the vegetables crunchy.

Prepare a large bowl of ice water and set aside. Bring a large saucepan of water to a boil over high heat. Lightly salt the water and add the vegetables. Cook just until the color of the vegetables is bright. Immediately drain in a colander and plunge into the ice water to stop the cooking. Drain well, season with salt and pepper to taste, and serve.

Roasting

Preheat the oven to 400 degrees F. In a bowl, toss the cut vegetables with enough extra virgin olive oil to coat them evenly. Transfer the vegetables to a baking sheet or low-sided roasting pan. Sprinkle lightly with salt, freshly ground black pepper, and your favorite dried herb(s), if desired. Roast, stirring occasionally, until easily pierced with the tip of a sharp knife and beginning to brown. Serve hot, at room temperature, or chilled.

Tips: If you want to roast several kinds of vegetables at the same time, keep them on separate baking sheets so that you can remove them from the oven as they're cooked. Roasted vegetables are especially good served with a drizzle of balsamic vinegar or a little Basic Vinaigrette (page 274).

THE FOOLPROOF GUIDE TO
COOKING VEGETABLES

| Vegetable | Size and Prep | Cooking Time in Minutes | | | | |
		Sauté	Steam	Boil	Blanch	Roast
Asparagus	Choose thin spears. Cut away and discard tough ends.	4–6	7–8	6–8	1–2	10–12
Beets	Choose small beets. *To sauté:* peel and shred. *To steam or boil:* leave whole and unpeeled. *To roast:* Combine whole, unpeeled beets with ¼ cup water in a tightly covered dish.	6–8	25–30	20–25		45–60
Bell peppers	Remove and discard seeds. Cut into thin strips.	5–7	—	—	1	20–25
Broccoli	Separate into small florets.	4–6	7–8	6–8	1–2	16–18
Cabbage — white, green, or red	Remove and discard the core. *To sauté:* shred. *To steam, boil, blanch, or roast:* cut into 1½-inch-thick wedges.	5–7	10–12	8–10	1–2	20–25
Carrots	Peel, if desired. *To sauté:* cut into thin slices. *To steam, boil, blanch, or roast:* cut into ½-inch chunks.	5–7	10–12	8–10	2–3	25–30

Vegetable	Size and Prep	Cooking Time in Minutes				
		Sauté	Steam	Boil	Blanch	Roast
Cauliflower	Separate into small florets.	4–6	7–9	7–9	1–2	15–18
Chard — green or red	Remove and discard any tough stems. Chop greens coarsely. Rinse well.	4–6*	4–6	4–6	1–2	—
Collard greens	Remove and discard any tough stems. Chop greens coarsely. Rinse well.	10–12*	10–12	10–12	2–3	—
Eggplant	Peel, if desired. Cut into 1-inch cubes or slices.	10–12	—	—	—	20–25
Green beans	Trim off and discard tough ends.	3–5	6–8	4–6	1–2	10–12
Kale	Remove and discard any tough stems. Chop greens coarsely. Rinse well.	8–10*	8–10	8–10	1–2	—
Mustard greens	Remove and discard any tough stems. Chop greens coarsely. Rinse well.	6–8*	6–8	6–8	1	—
Onions — sweet, yellow, white, or red	Peel. Thinly slice. *To roast:* cut into 1-inch-thick wedges.	8–10	10–12	8–10	2–3	35–40
Parsnips	Peel. Cut into ½-inch chunks.	—	13–15	12–14	—	35–45

Vegetable	Size and Prep	Cooking Time in Minutes				
		Sauté	Steam	Boil	Blanch	Roast
Peas	Remove from pods.	2–3	3–5	3–4	1	—
Rutabagas	Peel. Cut into ½-inch chunks.	—	16–18	14–16	—	35–45
Spinach	Chop coarsely. Rinse well.	3–5	4–6	3–5	1	—
Summer squash or zucchini	Cut into ¼-inch-thick slices.	5–7	5–7	5–7	1–2	20–30
Tomatoes	*To sauté:* Choose cherry tomatoes. Leave whole. *To roast:* Choose medium to large tomatoes. Cut in half and roast cut side up.	5–7	—	—	—	15–20
Turnips	Peel, if desired. Cut into ½-inch chunks.	—	12–14	10–12	2–3	30–35
Winter squash — butternut, acorn, kabocha, or buttercup	Peel. Cut in half to remove and discard seeds. Cut into 1-inch chunks.	—	14–16	12–14	—	30–35

*Add a few tablespoons of water, as described in the section on sautéing (see page 257).

The Foolproof Guide to Making Salads

A good salad can be so much more than a bowl of boring lettuce and bottled dressing — but that doesn't mean it has to be complicated or fancy.

Start with the greens. One generous cup of greens is about right for a single serving. Use just one type of greens or combine several. Romaine and iceberg lettuce, shredded cabbage, and bitter endive are crunchy choices; baby spinach and butter, green leaf, and red leaf lettuce are tenderer. You'll save money if you buy a whole head of lettuce and wash and dry it yourself. But you'll save time if you buy bags of prewashed salad greens.

A generous tablespoon of most vinaigrettes or dressings is usually ample for one serving of salad, but as long as you use healthful oils, there is no need to be stingy. If a little extra dressing will encourage your child to eat more veggies, go for it. Dressings can be as simple as a drizzle of extra virgin olive oil and vinegar (try red wine, rice wine, or balsamic vinegar). Add a little freshly squeezed lemon or orange juice to the mix for a citrus dressing. Take a few more minutes and add a couple of more ingredients, and you can have a delicious Basic Vinaigrette (page 274). With a minimum of effort, you can steer clear of the sugar, gums, preservatives, and artificial flavors in prepared bottled dressings.

The Foolproof Guide to Cooking Whole Grains

Whole grains have a reputation for being difficult and time-consuming to make. But many whole grains can be prepared in 30 to 40 minutes with little more effort than boiling a pot of water, and they're far more nutritious and filling than their refined cousins. Follow the package directions for cooking your whole grain of choice. If the directions are unclear or you buy in bulk, follow the table on page 264. For extra taste, drizzle cooked grains with extra virgin olive oil and season with salt, freshly ground black pepper, and/or savory herbs. All whole grains can be refrigerated or frozen, then reheated when needed to speed up weeknight dinner prep. A few whole grains, such as hulled barley and wheat berries, require presoaking to shorten cooking times, but you can put them in to soak in the morning so they're ready to cook for dinner.

To Cook Whole Grains That Don't Need Presoaking

Determine how much whole grain, water, and salt you need by referring to the table.

In a large, heavy-bottomed saucepan with a tight-fitting lid, bring the water to a boil over high heat. Stir in the whole grain and salt. Return to a boil, cover tightly, and reduce the heat to maintain a gentle boil. Cook until tender.

If there is still a bit of water left in the pan, remove the lid and cook for a minute or two longer to evaporate the water. Remove the pan from the heat and let rest, covered, for a few minutes. Fluff the grains with a fork and serve.

To Cook Whole Grains That Need Presoaking

Determine how much whole grain, water, and salt you need by referring to the table.

In a large, heavy-bottomed saucepan with a tight-fitting lid, combine the whole grain and water. Let soak for at least 4 hours or overnight. Bring the whole grain, soaking liquid, and salt to a boil over high heat. Cover tightly, reduce the heat to maintain a gentle boil, and proceed to cook as directed for grains that were not presoaked.

To Store Cooked Whole Grains

Allow the grain to cool, then transfer to airtight containers. (If you use 1-, 2-, or 4-cup containers, you can defrost just the amount you need later.) Refrigerate for up to 5 days or freeze for up to 1 month.

THE FOOLPROOF GUIDE TO COOKING WHOLE GRAINS

Yields about eight ½-cup servings

	Whole Grain	Water	Salt	Cooking Time
		Presoaking Not Required		
Brown rice*	1⅓ cups	2½ cups	½ teaspoon	About 50 min.
Wild rice	1 cup	2½ cups	½ teaspoon	About 1 hour
Pearl barley	1 cup	2½ cups	½ teaspoon	About 40 min.
Quinoa	1⅓ cups	2¼ cups	½ teaspoon	About 20 min.
Millet	1½ cups	3½ cups	½ teaspoon	About 30 min.
Amaranth	2 cups	3 cups	½ teaspoon	About 20 min.
		Presoaking Required		
Hulled barley	1¼ cups	3½ cups	½ teaspoon	Presoak: 4–12 hours Cook: About 50 min.
Wheat berries	2 cups	3¼ cups	½ teaspoon	Presoak: 4–12 hours Cook: About 50 min.

*Brown rice can be presoaked for 4–12 hours for a rich, nutty flavor.

The Foolproof Guide to Cooking Potatoes

To Bake Whole Potatoes, Sweet Potatoes, and Yams

Preheat the oven to 400 degrees F. Give the skins a good scrubbing under cold running water to remove any dirt. Using the tip of a sharp knife or a fork, pierce the skins in several places so they won't split as they bake. Place sweet potatoes and yams on aluminum foil or in a baking pan, as they can leak sugar as they bake. Bake until tender when pierced with the tip of a thin-bladed knife, about 1 hour. Cut open and season with salt and pepper to taste. Serve with a drizzle of extra virgin olive oil, if you like.

To Roast Cut Potatoes, Sweet Potatoes, and Yams

Preheat the oven to 400 degrees F. Cut the potatoes (peeled or unpeeled) into ½-inch-thick slices. Place in a baking dish just large enough to hold the potatoes in a single layer. Drizzle with enough extra virgin olive oil to lightly coat them. Season with salt and fresh or dried rosemary or thyme to taste. Roast, stirring occasionally, until golden brown and tender when pierced with the tip of a thin-bladed knife, 45 minutes to 1 hour depending on the variety and size. Serve.

Portion Proportions

Wondering how much protein, cooked vegetables, salad, and whole grains or potatoes to include in your balanced meal? You can eyeball the serving sizes by dividing your dinner plate into three sections (see Figure 9.2). Protein and whole grains or potatoes should each take up a quarter of your dinner plate. Cooked vegetables and salad should fill the remaining half. In weight or cup measures, these proportions translate to 3 to 4 ounces of protein, a moderate serving of whole grains or potatoes (1 slice of whole grain bread, ½ cup of cooked whole grains, or 3 ounces of potatoes), 1 cup of salad greens, and 1 or more cups of cooked vegetables.

Putting It All Together

The Mix-and-Match Basic Meal Planner and foolproof guides will get you started with the process of planning and cooking a simple, balanced, and tasty dinner. Once you get the hang of it, try chopping or cooking a little more of the basics on a night when you have some extra time (perhaps more vegetables and tofu on Sunday) to combine into another recipe when you are pressed for time. Whether you cook some basics ahead of time or start from scratch each day, the recipes below are creative ways to combine meal components into satisfying and healthful dinners.

❖ Spaghetti Veggie Medley

Yield: 6 servings

What kid doesn't like spaghetti? And what parent won't like the fact that this recipe is the perfect camouflage for a bunch of vegetables and whole grains. If you keep a few packages of whole grain pasta on hand in your pantry and some Basic Pasta and Pizza Sauce in your freezer or refrigerator, you'll have dinner in no time. Cut the prep time even more by using last night's leftover cooked veggies and chicken (toss them in at the last minute to reheat them). Substitute any of your favorite vegetables for the ones in the recipe — just keep in mind that harder vegetables such as cauliflower, broccoli, and carrots will take longer to cook than spinach and other leafy vegetables. If you prefer store-bought pasta sauce, buy a brand that doesn't list sugar as one of the first few ingredients.

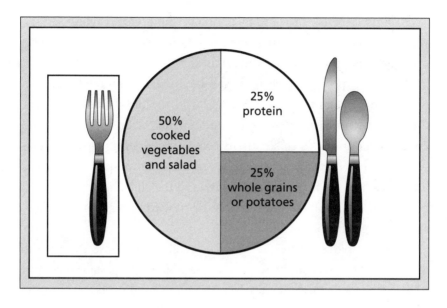

Figure 9.2 The Dinner Plate

Salt

1 pound whole grain spaghetti

1 tablespoon extra virgin olive oil

⅔ cup thinly sliced or small diced carrots

⅔ cup bite-size broccoli florets

⅔ cup thinly sliced or small diced zucchini and/or yellow summer squash

3 cups Basic Pasta and Pizza Sauce (page 280) or store-bought spaghetti sauce

1 cup diced cooked chicken, tempeh, or seitan

Freshly ground black pepper

1–2 tablespoons chopped fresh basil or parsley or 1–2 teaspoons dried basil or parsley

Freshly grated Parmesan cheese, for serving

Bring a large pot of water to a boil over high heat. Lightly salt the water and add the spaghetti. Cook according to the package directions until just tender. Drain well and set aside.

While the pasta is cooking, heat a large, wide-bottomed saucepan or soup pot over medium-high heat. Add the olive oil and carrots. Cook, stirring occasionally, for 4 minutes. Add the broccoli florets and zucchini. Continue to cook, stirring occasionally, until all the vegetables are just tender, about 3 minutes more. Add the pasta sauce and bring to a boil. Reduce the heat to low, add the chicken, and cook at a gentle simmer for about 5 minutes more to warm everything through and blend the flavors.

Add the pasta to the sauce and vegetables. Increase the heat to medium-high and cook, stirring occasionally, until the pasta absorbs just a bit of the sauce, 2 to 3 minutes. Season with salt and pepper to taste and stir in the basil. Serve hot, passing the grated Parmesan at the table.

TO ROUND OUT THE MEAL, serve with a dinner salad.

❖ Salad Bar Stir-Fry with Tofu or Chicken

Yield: 4 servings

A stir-fry is one of the quickest meals to prepare, and if you purchase the vegetables already sliced or chopped from your grocer's fresh salad bar, it's even faster. The three keys to a successful stir-fry are (1) to cut the tofu and vegetables into thin slices or bite-size pieces, (2) to use high heat, and (3) to keep tossing and stirring as you cook. That's it. Once you get the hang of stir-frying, experiment with other vegetable and flavor combinations. Use any vegetables you like, but try for an assortment of colors, flavors, and textures. Try Thai or teriyaki baked tofu, or add a handful of seeds or nuts. Broccoli and walnuts are especially good together, sesame seeds complement spinach, and chopped peanuts are nice sprinkled over most combinations.

Adding a little cornstarch at the end of the cooking will thicken the sauce, but it's really not necessary. If you want to use it, whisk it into the cold water just before you add the water to the pan. (Cornstarch tends to form lumps if you try to mix it into hot liquid, and it will settle to the bottom of the cup if you mix it into the water any sooner than you need it.)

2 tablespoons high-oleic safflower oil or extra virgin olive oil
1 pound savory baked tofu or 12 ounces cooked chicken, cut
  into matchsticks
1 cup thinly sliced yellow onion (1 onion)
1 cup bite-size broccoli florets
1 cup thinly sliced red bell pepper (1 pepper)
1 cup carrots sliced about ¼ inch thick (3 carrots)
1 cup snow peas
2 tablespoons finely minced garlic (4–5 cloves)
1 tablespoon peeled and minced fresh ginger
  (1-inch piece)
⅓ cup cold water
2 tablespoons soy sauce
1 tablespoon cornstarch (optional)
Salt and freshly ground black pepper
1–2 teaspoons toasted sesame oil (optional)
2 cups cooked brown rice, for serving

Garnishes (optional)
Thinly sliced green onions
Toasted sesame seeds

Heat a wok or large, heavy-bottomed skillet over high heat. Add 1 tablespoon of the safflower oil and swirl to coat the bottom of the pan. Add the tofu and cook, stirring, until it just begins to brown, about 3 minutes. Transfer to a small bowl and set aside.

Add the remaining 1 tablespoon safflower oil to the skillet. Swirl to coat the bottom of the pan. Add the onion, broccoli, pepper, carrots, and snow peas. Cook, stirring, until tender, 3 to 4 minutes. Return the tofu to the pan (or add the cooked chicken, if using). Stir in the garlic and ginger and cook until fragrant, 10 to 20 seconds. Add the water and soy sauce. If using the cornstarch, stir it into the water before adding to the pan. Cook, stirring, until the vegetables are glossy and the tofu is hot, about 2 minutes. Season with salt and pepper to taste. Drizzle with the sesame oil, if desired, and toss well.

Serve immediately over the rice. If you'd like, garnish with green onions and toasted sesame seeds.

❖ Hearty Barley, Vegetable, and Chicken Soup

Yield: 4 servings

You can make broth from scratch (you'll find recipes in almost any cookbook and hundreds online), but to save time, you can use good-quality canned or boxed broth. Look for a brand that's low sodium (so you can control how salty your soup is) and that doesn't have MSG, sugar, or artificial colors and flavors.

This soup comes together quickly if you have leftover barley or another whole grain (see page 264). The rest of the soup takes only about 15 minutes if you're using uncooked chicken and even less time if you're using leftover cooked chicken, tofu, or seitan.

6 cups chicken or vegetable broth
1 cup thinly sliced carrots
1 cup thinly sliced celery
2 cups cooked barley or other whole grain
12 ounces boneless, skinless chicken, cut into ½-inch chunks,

or 2 cups cooked chicken, extra-firm regular or savory
baked tofu, or seitan cut into ½-inch chunks
Salt and freshly ground black pepper
1 tablespoon chopped fresh parsley

In a soup pot or large saucepan, bring the broth to a boil over high heat. Add the carrots and celery, reduce the heat to low, and simmer gently, covered, until the vegetables are tender, about 4 minutes.

Add the barley and chicken. Simmer, stirring occasionally, until the chicken is no longer pink in the middle, 8 to 10 minutes. (If using cooked chicken, tofu, or seitan, cook until just heated through, 3 to 5 minutes.) Season with salt and pepper to taste, stir in the parsley, and serve.

TO ROUND OUT THE MEAL, serve with a dinner salad.

❖ Bean Chili

Yield: 4 servings

This chili can be pulled together quickly for dinner in less than an hour or cooked longer for a richer, more complex flavor. Chili just gets better with age. Use any beans you want: red kidney beans, red beans (chili beans), black beans, cannellini beans, great northern beans, pinto beans, even garbanzo beans. One type is delicious, but a mixture of several types will make your chili even more interesting in texture and flavor. Whether you cook your own beans or use canned, be sure to rinse them well under cold running water before using. The chili will keep, covered and refrigerated, for up to 1 week or frozen for several months. Freeze it in individual serving-size containers, and you'll have an instant meal when you need one. This recipe is easily doubled or tripled.

1 tablespoon extra virgin olive oil

2 cups minced yellow onions

1 heaping tablespoon minced garlic

2 tablespoons chili powder

1 tablespoon ground cumin

1 teaspoon dried oregano

Big pinch of red pepper flakes — if you like your chili spicy (optional)

4 cups canned beans (three 15-ounce cans), rinsed under cold running water and drained

4 cups canned small diced or crushed tomatoes with their juice (three 14.5-ounce cans)

1½ cups tempeh chopped or crumbled into small pieces (optional)

2 cups vegetable broth or water

Salt and freshly ground black pepper

Garnishes (optional)

Chopped fresh cilantro

Chopped green onions

Shredded cheddar or Monterey Jack cheese

Heat a soup pot or large saucepan over medium-high heat. When the pan is hot, add the oil. Add the onions and cook, stirring occasionally, until translucent and softened, about 5 minutes. Add the garlic and cook, stirring, until fragrant, about 1 minute. Add the chili powder, cumin, oregano, and red pepper flakes (if using). Stir until well combined. Add the beans, tomatoes with their juice, tempeh (if using), and broth. Reduce the heat to low and simmer gently, stirring occasionally, until the flavors have blended, about 30 minutes (or up to 1 hour for a richer, thicker chili). Season with salt and pepper to taste and serve hot. If desired, garnish with a generous sprinkling of cilantro, green onions, and shredded cheese.

TO ROUND OUT THE MEAL, serve with a dinner salad and warm corn tortillas.

❖ Chef's Salad

Yield: 4 servings

Another great-tasting, simple way to get most of the components of a healthy meal all together in one dish. Chef's salad was probably created to use up whatever meat, cheese, and vegetables the chef had sitting around in the refrigerator. And although last night's steamed or blanched veggies are perfectly good choices to use in your salad, the raw carrots, tomatoes, avocado, and bell pepper suggested here add great fresh flavors and crunch. You'll often find Thousand Island dressing or other creamy concoctions on a restaurant version of chef's salad, but the avocado and vinaigrette will give you all the creaminess without the chemicals, unhealthy fats, and artificial colors and flavors.

8 cups mixed salad greens or baby spinach

6 ounces cooked chicken or savory baked tofu, diced (about 1 cup), or 6 ounces sliced vegetarian cold cuts, cut into thin ribbons

4 ounces cheese (such as cheddar, Swiss, or Monterey Jack), grated, diced, or cut into matchsticks (about 1 cup)

2 large hard-boiled eggs, chopped or quartered

1 cup cherry tomatoes, halved

1 cup coarsely shredded carrots

1 cup diced avocado (1 large)

1 cup diced or thinly sliced bell pepper (red, yellow, orange, green, or a combination; about 1 pepper)

¼ cup Basic Vinaigrette (see next page) or extra virgin olive oil and vinegar for drizzling

Freshly ground black pepper

Arrange 2 cups of the salad greens on each of four dinner plates. Divide the chicken, cheese, eggs, carrots, tomatoes, avocado, and bell pepper among the plates, either scattering them over the greens or placing each in a separate pile or row on the greens. (You can also let the kids come up with their own designs.) Drizzle with the vinaigrette, add a few grinds of pepper, and serve.

TO ROUND OUT THE MEAL, serve with a cup of soup and a slice of whole grain bread.

BASIC VINAIGRETTE

Yield: ¼ cup

Vinaigrette is just the fancy French word for an oil and vinegar dressing, and it couldn't be simpler to make, easier to store, or more versatile to use. Five ingredients, plus salt and pepper, and you have one of the tastiest dressings you could put on a salad. Don't be tempted to skip the Dijon mustard or balsamic vinegar in this recipe. Dijon (rather than the standard yellow mustard) helps bind the oil and vinegar together and adds a less acidic mustard flavor. Balsamic vinegar rounds out the flavor and takes the edge off the finished dressing. If you like the taste of Italian-style dressings, you can add a big pinch of dried herbs: basil, oregano, marjoram, thyme, rosemary, sage, or a combination.

1 tablespoon red wine vinegar
½ teaspoon balsamic vinegar or ¼ teaspoon honey
½ teaspoon Dijon mustard
¼ teaspoon garlic powder

3 tablespoons extra virgin olive oil
Salt and freshly ground black pepper
Big pinch of dried herb(s) (see headnote; optional)

In a small jar, combine the red wine vinegar, balsamic vinegar, mustard, and garlic powder. Shake well to combine. Add the olive oil and shake vigorously until very well combined. (Alternatively, you can whisk the ingredients together in a small bowl.) Season with salt and pepper to taste, then add the herb(s), if using. The vinaigrette will keep, refrigerated, for at least 3 weeks.

❖ Fajitas

Yield: 4 servings

Fajitas are Mexican vaquero (cowboy) food. They're an easy stovetop dinner during the week or a festive party dinner for friends on the weekend.

Because this recipe cooks quickly, it's important to read it through before you start. Don't worry — you don't need to master any complicated methods or techniques; you just need to get a feel for the recipe. You may substitute more lime juice for the rice wine vinegar, if you like.

Marinade

¼ cup freshly squeezed lime juice

¼ cup rice wine vinegar

1 tablespoon extra virgin olive oil

1 tablespoon chopped green onions

1 tablespoon chopped fresh cilantro (optional)

1 teaspoon finely minced garlic

⅛ teaspoon dried oregano

Salt and freshly ground black pepper

12 ounces boneless, skinless chicken breasts, cut diagonally into ½-inch-wide strips, or 1 pound firm regular tofu or tempeh, cut into ½-inch-thick slices

Eight 7-inch whole grain tortillas

1 ripe avocado
1 tablespoon freshly squeezed lime juice

2 tablespoons extra virgin olive oil
2 cups thinly sliced bell peppers (a mixture of green, red,
    orange, and/or yellow is prettiest)
1 cup thinly sliced yellow onion
Salt and freshly ground black pepper

1 cup salsa, for serving

To make the marinade: In a medium, shallow dish or resealable plastic bag, combine the lime juice, vinegar, olive oil, green onions, cilantro (if using), garlic, oregano, and salt and pepper to taste. Stir or shake to mix. Add the chicken, cover the dish or seal the bag, and let marinate in the refrigerator for at least 20 minutes or up to 3 hours. When ready to cook, remove the chicken and pat dry with paper towels. Discard the marinade.

Heat the tortillas according to the package directions, or wrap the stack of tortillas in foil and place in a 250 degree F oven while you prepare the rest of the dinner.

Halve the avocado, remove and discard the pit, and scoop out the flesh. Thinly slice the avocado and arrange it on a small plate. Drizzle with the lime juice to keep it from turning brown and set aside.

Heat a large skillet over medium-high heat. Add 1 tablespoon of the oil and swirl to coat the bottom of the pan. Add the peppers and onion and cook, stirring occasionally, until just crisp-tender, 3 to 4 minutes. Season with salt and pepper to taste. Transfer to a bowl and keep warm.

Return the skillet to the heat. Add the remaining 1 tablespoon oil and swirl to coat the bottom of the pan. Add the marinated chicken and cook, stirring occasionally, for about 6 minutes, or until the chicken is no longer pink in the center. (If using tofu or tempeh, cook until golden brown on each side.)

Place the warm tortillas, sliced avocado, onion and peppers, chicken, and salsa where everyone can easily reach them. To assemble a fajita, place a tortilla on your plate. Add a spoonful of chicken, some of the onion and peppers, a spoonful of salsa, and a slice or two of avocado. Roll up and enjoy.

QUICK PICK!

❖ Pizza Anytime

Yield: 1 serving

This recipe offers pizza parlor flavor without the hassle of a complicated crust. And because you make each pizza individually, choosing your own combination of toppings, you can make 1 serving after basketball practice or 100 servings for a party.

For a bit of stealth nutrition, sneak a layer of mashed white beans under the cheese, next to the crust. Just rinse and drain canned beans, then mash them smooth with a fork. The texture of melted mozzarella and mashed beans is very similar, so you get the illusion of a cheesier pizza and the fiber of the beans. If you're short on time and want to use store-bought pizza sauce, look for one that has no added sugar or as little sugar as possible.

1 whole grain English muffin, split
¼ cup vegetable topping(s) (see page 279)
2 tablespoons shredded cheese
1 tablespoon protein topping (see page 279)
½ tablespoon chopped fresh basil or ½ teaspoon dried basil or
    Italian seasoning

½ teaspoon extra virgin olive oil

Salt and freshly ground black pepper

1 tablespoon mashed white beans (optional)

2 tablespoons Basic Pasta and Pizza Sauce (page 280) or store-
  bought pizza sauce

2 teaspoons freshly grated Parmesan cheese

Red pepper flakes (optional)

Preheat the oven or toaster oven to 350 degrees F. If you like your pizza extra-crispy, lightly toast the English muffin. Set aside.

In a small bowl, combine the vegetable topping(s), shredded cheese, protein topping, basil, and olive oil. Toss to combine. Season with salt and pepper to taste and set aside.

Spread each half of the English muffin with ½ tablespoon of the mashed white beans, if using, and 1 tablespoon of the pizza sauce. Divide the topping mixture between the muffin halves and sprinkle with the cheese. Place the pizzas on a baking sheet or in a baking dish. Bake until the cheeses have melted and the filling is hot, 5 to 7 minutes. Sprinkle with red pepper flakes, if using, and serve hot.

TO ROUND OUT THE MEAL, serve with a dinner salad.

PIZZA TOPPINGS

Mix and match these toppings or come up with your own.

Vegetables — diced or thinly sliced	Cheese	Protein
Artichoke hearts	Cheddar	Anchovies
Bell peppers	Feta	Chicken — smoked,
Broccoli	Goat	roasted, or
Eggplant — sautéed	Monterey Jack	barbecued
or roasted	Mozzarella	Ready-to-eat veggie
Garlic — fresh or roasted	Swiss	sausage
Green chiles		Savory baked tofu —
Jalapeños		any flavor
Mushrooms — fresh		Turkey — smoked,
or sautéed		roasted, or
Olives		barbecued
Onions		Veggie cold cuts
Tomatoes — fresh,		
roasted, or sun-dried		
Zucchini		

BASIC PASTA AND PIZZA SAUCE

Yield: 3 generous cups

Nothing ever tastes quite as good on pasta or pizza as homemade sauce. And when a recipe is as easy as this one, uses such inexpensive ingredients, and can be frozen so conveniently, you'll find yourself craving your own sauce more often.

Of course, great-tasting tomato sauce starts with great-tasting tomatoes, and canned tomatoes often result in a better sauce than fresh ones, which vary widely in quality and flavor. If your sauce is a bit too tart or acidic after it has simmered, add a little milk. The natural sugars present in milk will take the edge off the sauce.

Every Italian grandmother worth her *ragù* has a secret recipe for tomato sauce. Use this one as a guideline, adding a little more garlic here or a little less basil there, and you can create your own "old family recipe."

1 tablespoon extra virgin olive oil
1 cup finely diced yellow onion
2–3 teaspoons finely minced garlic
One 28-ounce can crushed tomatoes with their juice
1 cup vegetable broth or water
1 bay leaf
2 teaspoons dried basil or Italian seasoning
1 teaspoon dried oregano or Italian seasoning
Big pinch of red pepper flakes (optional)
2–3 tablespoons milk (if needed)
Salt and freshly ground black pepper

Heat a large saucepan over medium-high heat. When the pan is hot, add the oil. Add the onion and cook, stirring occasionally, until translucent and tender, about 5 minutes. Add the garlic and cook, stirring, until fragrant, about 1 minute. Add the tomatoes and their juice, the broth, bay leaf, basil, oregano, and red pepper flakes (if using). Stir until well combined. Bring to a boil, reduce the heat to low, and simmer gently, stirring occasionally, until the flavors have blended and the tomatoes have broken down into a thick saucelike consistency, about 20 minutes. (If you have time, the sauce will taste even better if you let it simmer slowly for another 20 to 30 minutes. Just watch that it doesn't get too thick and start to scorch on the bottom of the pan. If it seems like it might, you can add a bit more broth or water.)

After simmering, taste the sauce. If it seems a little too acidic or tart, add the milk. Season with salt and pepper to taste.

Use immediately or let cool to room temperature before transferring to airtight containers. The sauce will keep in the refrigerator for up to 5 days or in the freezer for several months.

Sweet Endings

Most cultures around the world end the main meal of the day with some fresh seasonal fruit, a little cheese, or even just a cup of hot herbal tea, saving the fancy, elaborate cookies, cakes, and candies to celebrate special occasions and holidays.

Unfortunately, we Americans either overdo the desserts or deny ourselves completely — making us feel terribly guilty or totally deprived. Actually, dessert can help us avoid overeating by bringing the meal to a timely close. Plus, it tastes good. Keep in mind, the goal of dessert is to provide a touch of something refreshing, rich, or sweet after a balanced meal — not the day's calorie requirement in one dish. Any way you slice it, a 1,500-calorie banana split is a recipe for trouble. So let's restore dessert to its rightful place as a "de-LITE-ful" way to end dinner.

The following recipes offer a sweet, but not too sweet, ending to your meal, ranging from hot drinks such as cocoa to baked treats such as apple crisp. Some are a bit exotic, such as masala chai, a spice-infused milky tea. Others are familiar favorites, such as rice pudding, with a healthy twist. We guarantee that you'll find something to please just about any dessert craving.

QUICK PICK!

❖ Hot Herbal Tea

Yield: 1 serving

A cup of fragrant, hot herbal tea after dinner is the easiest way to end a meal on a pleasant note. Aromatic mint or licorice teas are especially popular with kids, but any herbal tea is fine.

1 cup cold water
1 bag herbal tea
1–2 teaspoons honey (optional)

In a kettle or small saucepan, bring the water to a boil over high heat. Place the tea bag in a large mug or teacup. Immediately pour the boiling water over the tea and let steep for 3 to 4 minutes. Remove and discard the tea bag, sweeten with honey (if desired), and enjoy.

❖ Masala Chai

Yield: 1 serving

Masala chai is Hindi for "spiced tea." This milky, spice-infused tea so popular in India (and now much of the rest of the world) is both a lovely way to start the day and a relaxing way to end it.

Every recipe for masala chai is a little bit different, so don't be afraid to experiment. Try just one spice, such as cardamom, for a very mellow, sweet tea. Leave out a spice in the masala if you don't care for it, or substitute one you like better. If you don't want to mix your own spices, look for premade chai tea at your local grocery store. Some stores even carry heat-and-serve masala chai in shelf-stable boxes.

1 cup cold water
½ cup low-fat milk or soy milk
½ teaspoon Masala (recipe follows)
2 bags black tea (such as English Breakfast tea), regular or de-caffeinated
2 teaspoons pure maple syrup, honey, or agave nectar (see page 223; optional)

In a small saucepan, bring the water and milk to a boil. Add the masala and tea bags, remove from the heat, and let steep, covered, for 4 minutes. Remove the tea bags. Stir in the maple syrup, if desired, and serve hot.

Masala (Spice Powder)

This makes enough for 5 to 6 servings of masala chai. If you like, the recipe can easily be doubled or quadrupled.

1 teaspoon ground cardamom
1 teaspoon ground cinnamon
½ teaspoon ground ginger
¼ teaspoon ground cloves
⅛ teaspoon freshly ground black pepper

In a small container with a tight-fitting lid, combine the cardamom, cinnamon, ginger, cloves, and pepper. Shake to mix well. Store in a cool, dark cupboard for up to 4 months.

❖ Drinking Chocolate

Yield: 1 serving

This is not your ordinary cup of hot cocoa. Unsweetened cocoa powder is dissolved in hot water and sweetened with a bit of maple syrup and vanilla extract. The flavor is intensely chocolate and only slightly sweet — more like the drink of the ancient Maya and Aztecs (only without the ground chiles). Hershey, Nestlé, and Droste all make unsweetened cocoa powder, and there are also very good organic cocoas on the market if you want to seek them out.

1½ tablespoons unsweetened cocoa powder
1 tablespoon pure maple syrup, honey, or agave nectar (see page 223)

⅛ teaspoon vanilla extract

1 cup boiling water

In a mug or large coffee cup, combine the cocoa powder, maple syrup, and vanilla extract. Add an inch or so of the boiling water and stir well to dissolve. Add the rest of the boiling water. Stir and serve hot.

QUICK PICK!

❖ Fresh Fruit

Many cultures around the world (the Italians, Chinese, and French, to name just a few) like to end their main meal with fruit. Fresh seasonal fruit is naturally sweet, fragrant, and satisfying, and it's one of the easiest things to serve for dessert. Let the calendar be your guide.

Select fruit that is at its best for the season — apples, pears, and pineapple in the winter; peaches, apricots, plums, and cherries in the summer. Choose one type of fruit or a combination. Wash, peel, seed, core, and cut the fruit into wedges or bite-size pieces. Arrange in a bowl or on a platter. Or mix different chopped fruits together and portion into individual serving bowls. Drizzle with a bit of honey or maple syrup, if you like, or add some chopped dates. Enjoy your sweet ending to the day.

❖ Berries, Yogurt, and Honey

Yield: 4 servings

A bowl of fresh berries, yogurt, and honey is a light treat at the end of a meal. Combine several different kinds of berries or use just one or two, but make sure all are at their peak of flavor and ripeness. Be gentle when dealing with fresh berries, as they are fragile. Try to use them the same day you buy them.

> 3 cups fresh berries (such as raspberries, blueberries, strawberries, and/or blackberries)
> 1 tablespoon plus 1 teaspoon honey
> ¼ cup plain low-fat yogurt
> ⅛ teaspoon vanilla extract

Just before you are ready to assemble the dessert, place the berries in a colander and rinse under cold running water. Transfer to a medium bowl, drizzle with 1 tablespoon of the honey, and toss gently to coat.

In a small bowl, combine the yogurt, the remaining 1 teaspoon honey, and the vanilla extract. Mix well.

Divide the berries among four bowls. Top each with a tablespoon of the honey-vanilla yogurt and serve.

❖ Baked Peaches

Yield: 4 servings

When you find that perfectly ripe peach, sit down and enjoy it just as nature gave it to you. But for those more common, still-a-bit-too-firm grocery store peaches and nectarines, try baking them. Baking concentrates the flavor and sweetness of the fruit and softens the flesh. Here, crunchy sliced almonds provide a nice contrast in texture and flavor. Or add a dollop of almond yogurt for a spectacular dessert.

> 4 firm, ripe peaches or nectarines
> 1 teaspoon maple syrup or honey
>
> *Almond Yogurt (optional)*
> ½ cup plain low-fat yogurt

1 tablespoon pure maple syrup or honey

3 drops almond extract

2–3 tablespoons toasted sliced almonds (see page 211)

Preheat the oven to 350 degrees F. Lightly oil a baking dish just large enough to hold the peach halves in a single layer.

Cut the peaches in half and discard the pits. Place the peaches cut side up in the baking dish. Brush (or use your fingertip to paint) a light coating of maple syrup over the cut surfaces. (If you have trouble getting the fruit to come off the pit easily, cut the fruit off the pit in thick slices and toss with the maple syrup before placing in the baking dish.)

Bake until hot and very tender when pierced with the tip of a small, sharp knife, 20 to 25 minutes.

Meanwhile, make the almond yogurt, if using. In a small bowl, combine the yogurt, honey, and almond extract. Mix well. Refrigerate until ready to serve.

Serve the baked fruit hot, warm, or at room temperature with a dollop of almond yogurt (if using) and a sprinkling of toasted almonds.

QUICK PICK!

❖ Nuts and Dried Fruit

A handful of nuts still in their shells (walnuts, pecans, almonds, hazelnuts, or macadamia nuts) and a few pieces of dried fruit (apricots, cherries, plums, or figs) are a great choice for dessert. Sit down with your family and friends while you crack the nuts, and you will find that you eat less and enjoy them more. Nutcrackers can be found in many grocery stores or hardware stores. You can find nuts still in their shells in most grocery stores during the fall and winter months.

❖ Sautéed Apple Crisp

Yield: 4 servings

No need to heat up the oven — this stovetop twist on apple crisp couldn't be easier or quicker to make, even on a busy weeknight. Use tart green apples such as Granny Smiths or Newtown Pippins for a bright apple flavor.

    2 teaspoons high-oleic safflower oil
    4 tart green apples, peeled, cored, and cut into small chunks
    1 tablespoon pure maple syrup
    ½ cup granola

Heat the oil in a medium skillet over medium heat. Add the apples and cook, stirring often, until golden brown and beginning to soften, 3 to 5 minutes. Add the maple syrup and continue to cook until the apples are tender when pierced with the tip of a small, sharp knife, 3 to 5 minutes more.

Divide the hot apples among four bowls (or take the skillet to the table and serve them straight from the pan). Sprinkle 2 tablespoons of the granola over each serving and serve.

❖ Maple Rice Pudding

Yield: 4 servings

Just three ingredients and 45 minutes will give you some serious comfort food. Keep some cooked brown rice in the freezer, and you can make this creamy pudding whenever the mood strikes.

    2 cups cooked brown rice
    3 cups plain rice milk, soy milk, or low-fat milk

2–3 tablespoons pure maple syrup, honey, or agave nectar (see
    page 223)
Ground cinnamon, for garnish (optional)

In a medium saucepan, combine the rice, rice milk, and maple
syrup. Stir to combine. Bring to a boil, reduce the heat to medium-low,
and simmer, uncovered and stirring occasionally, until the pudding is
thick, about 45 minutes. (If you draw a spoon through the pudding,
you will see the bottom of the pan for a second or two before the pudding settles over the bottom again.) Remove from the heat. Serve hot,
warm, at room temperature, or chilled, garnished with a sprinkling of
ground cinnamon, if desired.

❖ Sweet Potato Pie

Yield: One 9-inch pie or six ½-cup custards

Holidays and special occasions deserve a slightly more elaborate dessert. This creamy, custardy pie fits the bill perfectly. Start with whole
wheat graham crackers (found at natural food stores) for the crispy,
toasty crust. Avoid the brands with partially hydrogenated (trans) fats
and concentrated sweeteners such as high-fructose corn syrup. For a
fast, low-tech way to grind the crackers into crumbs, place the whole
crackers in a resealable plastic bag and whack and roll over it with a
rolling pin. (Your kids will love doing this.) To make this recipe even
easier, skip the graham cracker crust and bake the filling in ovenproof
custard cups. Serve the custards with a graham cracker on the side.

2 medium sweet potatoes (about 1 pound)

Graham Cracker Crust (optional)
2 tablespoons high-oleic safflower oil
1½ tablespoons water, plus more if needed

1 tablespoon pure maple syrup or honey

1⅔ cups finely ground whole wheat graham crackers

Sweet Potato Filling

2 large eggs, lightly beaten, or ½ cup liquid egg substitute

¾ cup buttermilk

¼ cup pure maple syrup

1 teaspoon vanilla extract

1 teaspoon ground cinnamon

⅛ teaspoon ground allspice

⅛ teaspoon ground nutmeg

Pinch of salt

¼ cup toasted pecan halves (see page 211), for garnish

To prepare the sweet potatoes: Preheat the oven to 425 degrees F. Line a baking sheet with aluminum foil. Prick the potatoes several times with a fork and place on the baking sheet. Bake until very tender, about 45 minutes. Let cool completely. Peel off the skins, transfer the flesh to a bowl, and mash until very smooth. Set aside 1½ cups for the filling. Save any leftovers for another use. (The potatoes can be prepared up to this point 1 day ahead and stored, covered, in the refrigerator. Return to room temperature before proceeding.)

Preheat the oven to 350 degrees F. Lightly oil a 9-inch pie plate; set aside.

To make the crust: In a medium bowl, combine the oil, water, and maple syrup. Mix well. Add the ground graham crackers and toss well to coat. The mixture should feel like damp sand and hold together when you pinch a small amount between your fingertips. If it doesn't, sprinkle another teaspoon or so of water over the mixture and toss to combine. Transfer to the prepared pie plate. Using lightly oiled hands, press the crumbs firmly into an even layer over the bottom and up the sides of the pie plate.

Bake for 7 minutes. The crust will feel a bit soft when it's hot but will firm and crisp up as it cools. Let cool completely. (The crust can be prepared up to this point 1 day ahead and stored, wrapped in plastic wrap, at room temperature.)

Preheat the oven to 350 degrees F.

To make the filling: In a large bowl, combine the mashed sweet potatoes and eggs. Mix well. Add the buttermilk, maple syrup, vanilla, cinnamon, allspice, nutmeg, and salt. Mix well again. If using the pie crust, pour the filling into the cooled crust. If baking without the crust, oil six ½-cup ovenproof custard cups and divide the filling among them.

Bake until the filling is just set and a thin-bladed, sharp knife inserted in the center comes out clean, 40 to 50 minutes for the pie or about 30 minutes for the custards. Let cool completely, about 1 hour, then cover with plastic wrap and refrigerate until firm and cold, 3 to 4 hours. When ready to serve, garnish with the toasted pecan halves. Cut the pie into wedges or serve the custards in their cups.

❖ Oatmeal, Walnut, and Apricot Cookies

Yield: 2 dozen cookies

These cookies are loaded with chewy oatmeal, crunchy walnuts, and sweet-tart dried apricots. The applesauce gives them a tender, soft, puffy texture, almost like a muffin top. Don't hesitate to substitute pecans, almonds, or other nuts for the walnuts, or dried apples, raisins, or dried cranberries for the apricots.

Two things will make baking these cookies easier: insulated baking sheets and parchment paper. Insulated baking sheets have a layer or "cushion" of air inside that keeps the bottoms of cookies from burning. You'll find them in most mass retail stores and housewares stores. Parchment paper keeps cookies from sticking without greasing the pan, and cleanup is a breeze. You can find it in the grocery store, next to the aluminum foil and plastic wrap.

¾ cup whole wheat flour

½ cup rolled oats (not instant or quick-cooking)

1 teaspoon baking soda

1 teaspoon ground cinnamon

¼ teaspoon salt

½ cup unsweetened smooth applesauce

¼ cup high-oleic safflower oil

¼ cup pure maple syrup

1 large egg, lightly beaten, or ¼ cup liquid egg substitute

1 teaspoon vanilla extract

½ cup chopped dried apricots

½ cup chopped toasted walnuts (see page 211)

Preheat the oven to 350 degrees F. Line two baking sheets with parchment paper or oil the baking sheets lightly.

In a large bowl, combine the flour, oats, baking soda, cinnamon, and salt. Stir well to mix. In a medium bowl, combine the applesauce, oil, maple syrup, egg, and vanilla. Whisk to combine. Pour the applesauce mixture into the flour mixture and stir just until the dry ingredients are moistened. Stir in the apricots and walnuts.

Drop heaping tablespoons of the dough onto the prepared baking sheets, leaving 1½ inches between the mounds. Bake until lightly browned and firm to the touch, 10 to 12 minutes. Let cool for a few minutes on the baking sheets before transferring to a wire rack to cool completely.

The cookies can be stored in an airtight container at room temperature for up to 3 days or frozen for up to 1 month.

Snack Attack

Snacking is a healthy part of a balanced diet — if you make the right choices. Use the following suggestions, and you'll be ready with a winning strategy when hunger sneaks up on you.

Plan ahead: Prepare snacks in advance so you'll have a healthy alternative to junk food when hunger strikes. Try fresh fruit, cut-up veggies and dips, or trail mix. Have your kids tuck a little healthy snack into their backpacks or pockets to protect against the pull of those vending machines and mini-marts.

Pay attention to hunger: Are you (or is your child) truly hungry or just bored? Will you be eating dinner in an hour, and if so, will something small suffice? Or is dinner several hours away, and you need something more substantial?

Keep it simple: Set aside a drawer or cupboard in your kitchen and a shelf in your refrigerator as "no thinking needed" snack zones. Fill them with simple, ready-to-eat (or nearly assembled) healthy snacks. The following suggestions will give you a good head start on filling those zones with healthy options.

Fruits and Veggies

- QUICK PICK! Use a bowl of assorted (washed) fruit as the centerpiece of your kitchen. Make it easy for your family to reach for a healthy snack without a second thought.
- Keep cut melon, berries, and other ready-to-eat fruits in separate containers, front and center, in the refrigerator. Give the berries and fruits a rinse under cold running water just before eating.
- Arrange raw or blanched vegetables (see page 258) on a pretty platter and keep it in the refrigerator. Add a few containers of

dips (see below), and you can have veggies and dip any time. (The veggies will keep for several days if tightly wrapped.)

Nuts and Crunch

- Trail mix can be as simple as combining a handful of nuts and a handful of dried fruit in a small resealable plastic bag. Make a few extra bags and stash one in your kid's backpack for a last-minute snack.
- Craving crunch? Make your own pita chips. Cut whole grain pita breads in half lengthwise so you have two flat rounds. Brush the rough side of the pitas lightly with extra virgin olive oil (optional). Cut into wedges and arrange rough side up on a large baking sheet. If you like, sprinkle with salt, pepper, dried or fresh herbs, and/or freshly grated Parmesan cheese. Bake in a preheated 400 degree F oven until lightly browned and crisp, 6 to 8 minutes. These chips are great served with soups and salads, too.
- Nutrition bars are very portable and keep well, but read the labels: many are more cookie than health bar. Choose one with at least 10 grams of protein.

Spreads and Dip

- Take a trip around the world just by visiting your grocer's refrigerator section. Browse the offerings of fresh spreads, dips, and salsas: garlicky hummus from the Middle East; creamy, crunchy yogurt and cucumber dip from Greece; salsas and guacamoles from Mexico. Spread your favorites on whole grain crackers or toast for a satisfying snack, or serve with raw vegetables. Don't forget peanut butter and other nut butters, too.
- You can make two quick dips of your own — savory for veggies and sweet for fruits. For a savory dip: season plain low-fat yogurt with salt, pepper, chopped fresh or dried herbs, and very finely minced garlic or onion. For a sweet dip: season plain low-fat yo-

gurt with a bit of maple syrup or honey and a few drops of vanilla or almond extract.

... Plus a Few More

- QUICK PICK! Store hard-boiled eggs in the refrigerator (for up to 5 days), and you'll have a peel-and-eat snack in a second. Or slice the eggs and use them to top a piece of whole grain toast spread with a little mayonnaise. Just season the eggs with salt and pepper to taste. Don't forget to mark the hard-boiled eggs for quick identification in the refrigerator.
- Cut tart apples or ripe pears crosswise into ¼-inch-thick slices. Use the sharp tip of a paring knife or a tiny round cookie cutter to remove the center core and seeds from each slice . Place a slice of cheddar cheese between two slices of fruit for a unique sandwich.
- Plain cottage cheese becomes a sweet treat if you stir in some diced fresh fruit or a dollop of all-fruit jam. Or season the cottage cheese with salt, pepper, dried or fresh herbs, and finely sliced green onions for a savory spread to use on whole grain crackers or toast.
- Smoothies make cool and refreshing energy boosters. Try our Silky Berry-Bursting Smoothie on page 224. If the eye-popping purple color doesn't give you a boost, the healthy combination of fruit and yogurt surely will.

❖ **PART VI** ❖

Reinforcements

DIARIES FOR THE
9-WEEK PROGRAM

Instructions for the Diaries

The Preparation Diary and the Weekly Diary are designed to guide you through the 9-Week Program. Each diary extends over two adjacent pages. After making copies for each family member, tape or staple the adjacent pages together for ease of use. (Copies are also available at www.endingthefoodfight.com.)

Preparation Diary

- The Preparation Diary is used during preparation week only. It is designed to help you take stock of your habits. The Behaviors column lists twenty-four key diet or physical activity behaviors, such as servings of vegetables eaten or hours of TV viewed per day. (Note that TV viewing is counted as part of screen time and also by itself.) At the end of each day during preparation week, family members record behaviors in their diaries. We suggest that this be done together as a family for support.
- At the end of preparation week, add up the numbers for each be-

havior throughout the week and record the total in the Weekly Total column.

- For those behaviors measured per day, divide by 7 as indicated and enter this number in the Typical Habits column. A calculator will be helpful. Note that some behaviors, such as having breakfast, are recorded simply as yes or no. For these behaviors, add up the number of yeses during the week and record that number in the Weekly Total column. As indicated by the ⇒, you will carry this number over to the Typical Habits column.

Weekly Diary

- After completing preparation week, transfer the numbers from the Typical Habits column of the Preparation Diary into the Typical Habits column of the Weekly Diary.
- Over the next nine weeks, you will "Step Up" or "Step Down" these behaviors to meet the targets listed in the Goal and Program Points column. For example, in Week 1 the vegetable goal is 4 servings a day for big kids and adults. For a teenager whose Typical Habit is 1 serving a day, Step Up to 2 servings on Monday, 3 servings on Tuesday, and 4 servings on Wednesday, then continue 4 servings a day for the rest of the week. Also in Week 1, the total screen time goal is 2 hours a day. For a family member whose Typical Habit is 6 hours a day, Step Down to 5 hours on Monday, 4 hours on Tuesday, 3 hours on Wednesday, and 2 hours on Thursday, then continue at 2 hours a day (maximum) for the rest of the week. If you already meet a specific goal for the week, keep it up and give yourself a pat on the back!
- During each successive week of the program, you will focus on a different set of behaviors. As you end one week and move to the next, try to maintain the behaviors you previously learned. However, you will monitor only those behaviors highlighted for that week in the Weekly Diary. For example, you will stop recording vegetables, fruits, and screen time when Week 2 begins, and start recording breakfasts, refined grains, and walking.

• Program Points are earned by reaching the goals for each week's highlighted behaviors. Record the number of Program Points earned each week in the Points Earned column. Note that keeping an accurate record of each behavior in the Weekly Diary earns 1 Program Point, whether or not you reached that goal. Bonus Points can be earned for some behaviors. Keep a running tally of Program Points in the Weekly Total column and let your kids know when they have accumulated enough for a reward.

Now, let's get with the program!

GUIDE TO SERVING SIZE

❖ Refer to this guide as you monitor and record your intake of various foods during preparation week and the 9-Week Program that follows.

Food	Serving Size
Fruit	1 medium fruit ½ cup fruit salad
Vegetable	1 cup raw ½ cup cooked
Bread	1 slice
Cereal (dry)	About 1 cup (see nutrition facts label)
Cereal (hot)	About ½ cup cooked (see nutrition facts label)
Grain (rice, pasta, etc.)	½ cup cooked
Beans/legumes	½ cup cooked
Vegetarian protein (veggie cold cuts, tofu, tempeh, seitan)	4 ounces
Fish/chicken	3 ounces
Nuts	⅓ cup
Nut butters	2 tablespoons
Eggs	1 egg or 2 egg whites
Cheese (hard)	1 ½ ounces

PREPARATION DIARY

Name of Family Member: _____

Start Date: _____

Behaviors	Mon.	Tues.	Wed.	Thurs.
Vegetables — excluding corn and potatoes (# servings a day)				
Fruits (# servings a day)				
Screen time — TV, video, computer for recreation (# hours a day)				
Breakfast (Y/N)				
Refined grains — white bread, white rice, etc. (# servings a day)				
Walking (# minutes a day)				
Home-prepared lunch (Y/N)				
Juice — 100% only (# cups a day)				
Sugary drinks (# cups a day)				
Water or no-calorie beverages (# cups a day)				
NEAT Activities — see page 162 (# a day)				
Vegetarian protein — see page 164 (# servings a day)				
Red meat (# servings a day)				
Active play — see page 165 (At least 30 min., Y/N)				
Healthy snacks — see page 168 (Was at least one healthy snack eaten? Y/N)				
Trans fats — see page 169 (# foods with trans fats a day)				
Active sports — see page 169 (At least 30 min., Y/N)				
Balanced meals — containing protein, low-glycemic carbohydrate, and healthy fat (# a day)				
Active travel — walk, bike, scooter, skateboard, etc. (Y/N)				
Healthy dessert after dinner — see page 174 (Y/N)				
Sugary treats (# a day)				
Active chore (Y/N)				
Eating out — salad, nonstarchy veggie, or fruit with every meal/snack eaten out (Y/N)				
TV (**# hours a day**)				

Fri.	Sat.	Sun.	Weekly Total	Typical Habits (daily or weekly average)
				÷ 7 = _____ servings of vegetables a day
				÷ 7 = _____ servings of fruits a day
				÷ 7 = _____ hour screen time a day
				⇒ _____ days a week eating breakfast
				÷ 7 = _____ servings of refined grains a day
				÷ 7 = _____ minutes of walking a day
				⇒ _____ days a week eating a home-prepared lunch
				÷ 7 = _____ cups of juice a day
				÷ 7 = _____ cups of sugary drinks a day
				÷ 7 = _____ cups of water or no-calorie beverages a day
				⇒ _____ number of NEAT activities a week
				÷ 7 = _____ servings of vegetarian protein a day
				÷ 7 = _____ servings of red meat a day
				⇒ _____ days a week with at least 30 minutes of active play
				⇒ _____ days a week with at least one healthy snack
				÷ 7 = _____ foods with trans fats a day
				⇒ _____ days a week with at least 30 minutes of active sports
				÷ 7 = _____ balanced meals a day
				⇒ _____ days a week using active travel
				⇒ _____ days a week having a healthy dessert after dinner
				⇒ _____ sugary treats a week
				⇒ _____ days a week with an active chore
				⇒ _____ days a week with a salad, veggie, or fruit if eating out
				÷ 7 = _____ hours of TV a day

WEEKLY DIARY

Name of Family Member: _____

Start Date: _____

	Behaviors	Typical Habits (from Preparation Diary)	Mon.	Tues.	Wed.	Thurs.
WEEK 1	Vegetables	_____ servings a day				
	Fruits	_____ servings a day				
	Screen time	_____ hours a day				
WEEK 2	Breakfast (Y/N)	_____ days a week				
	Refined grains	_____ servings a day				
	Walking	_____ minutes a day				
WEEK 3	Homemade lunch (Y/N)	_____ days a week				
	Juice	_____ cups a day				
	Sugary drinks	_____ cups a day				
	Water/no-calorie drinks	_____ cups a day				
	NEAT activities	_____ times a week				
WEEK 4	Vegetarian protein	_____ servings a day				
	Red meat	_____ servings a day				
	Active play (Y/N)	_____ days a week				
WEEK 5	Healthy snacks (Y/N)	_____ days a week				
	Trans fats	_____ foods a day				
	Active sports (Y/N)	_____ days a week				
WEEK 6	Balanced meals	_____ times a day				
	Active travel (Y/N)	_____ days a week				
WEEK 7	Healthy dessert (Y/N)	_____ days a week				
	Sugary treats (Y/N)	_____ times a week				
	Active chore (Y/N)	_____ days a week				
WEEK 8	Salad, vegetable, or fruit—eating out (Y/N)	_____ days a week				
	TV Turnoff (Y/N)	_____ hours a day				
WEEK 9	Choice to Step Up					
	Choice to Step Down					

Name of Family Member: _____

Start Date: _____

Fri.	Sat.	Sun.	Goal and Program Points	Points Earned	Weekly Total
			3 servings a day for little kids = 1 point 4 servings a day for big kids and adults = 1 point		
			2 servings a day for little kids = 1 point 3 servings a day for big kids and adults = 1 point		Monitoring: Add 1 pt. Total _____
			No more than 2 hours a day = 1 point BONUS: 10 hrs. screen time max this week = 1 point		
			Every day = 1 point		
			No more than 3 servings a day = 1 point		Monitoring: Add 1 pt. Total _____
			30 minutes a day = 1 point BONUS: walk at least 1 hour on 1 day = 1 point		
			4 days a week = 1 point		
			No more than 1 cup a day = 1 point		
			Zero = 1 point		
			At least 5 cups a day for little kids = 1 point At least 7 cups a day for big kids and adults = 1 point		Monitoring: Add 1 pt. Total _____
			7 times this week = 1 point		
			3 servings a day = 1 point BONUS: 1 day completely vegetarian = 1 point		
			Zero = 1 point		Monitoring: Add 1 pt. Total _____
			4 days a week for 30 minutes = 1 point		
			1–3 a day = 1 point		
			Zero = 1 point		Monitoring: Add 1 pt. Total _____
			3 days a week for 30 minutes = 1 point		
			2 a day = 1 point BONUS: 3 balanced meals every day = 2 points		Monitoring: Add 1 pt. Total _____
			Every day = 1 point		
			Every day = 1 point		
			No more than once this week = 1 point		Monitoring: Add 1 pt. Total _____
			5 days a week = 1 point		
			Every snack/meal away from home = 2 points BONUS: no fast food all week = 2 points		Monitoring: Add 1 pt. Total _____
			No TV all week = 3 points		
			Met goal = 1 point		Monitoring: Add 1 pt. Total _____
			Met goal = 1 point		

SHOPPING LIST

In the Fridge

Beverages
- Any beverage with 10 calories or less per serving
- 100 percent fruit juice (6 ounces per day maximum)
- Low-fat milk
- Seltzer or mineral water (unsweetened)
- Soy milk (plain)
- Vegetable juice (e.g., V8)
- Water

Condiments and Dressings
- Crushed garlic
- Ginger
- Ketchup (check to make sure sugar or corn syrup isn't one of the first few ingredients)
- Mayonnaise
- Mustard

- Pesto
- Preserves (with fruit, not sugar, listed as first ingredient)
- Salad dressing (regular, not fat-free)
- Salsa

Cheese and Yogurt
- Cottage cheese (regular)
- Hard cheese, regular or low fat (e.g., cheddar, Jack, Parmesan)
- Plain yogurt (low fat)
- String cheese

Dips and Spreads (all-natural, no sugar added)
- Almond butter
- Bean dip
- Cashew butter
- Guacamole
- Hummus
- Peanut butter
- Sour cream

Eggs
- Eggs
- Liquid egg substitute

Fruits
- Apples
- Apricots
- Blackberries
- Blueberries
- Cantaloupe
- Cherries
- Clementines
- Grapefruit
- Grapes

- Kiwifruit
- Nectarines
- Oranges
- Peaches
- Pears
- Plums
- Raspberries
- Strawberries

Protein

- Fish (e.g., cod, sardines, tuna, wild salmon) *Note:* Because of tuna's moderately high mercury content, limit it to once a week.
- Poultry (chicken and turkey)
- Shellfish (crab, scallops, shrimp)
- Vegetarian protein (tofu, tempeh, seitan, vegetarian cold cuts)

Vegetables (nonstarchy)

- Artichokes
- Asparagus
- Avocados
- Broccoli
- Cabbage
- Carrots
- Cauliflower
- Celery
- Collard greens
- Eggplant
- Green beans
- Kale
- Lettuce
- Mushrooms
- Mustard greens
- Okra
- Onions

- Peppers
- Spinach
- Summer squash (yellow crookneck and zucchini)
- Tomatoes

In the Freezer

Fruits (no sugar added)
- Blueberries
- Mixed berries
- Strawberries

Protein
- Ground turkey or chicken
- Shrimp and other seafood
- Soy (e.g., burgers, crumbles, dogs)

Vegetables
- Broccoli
- Cauliflower
- Green beans
- Peppers
- Stir-fry mix

In the Pantry

Canned Foods
- Artichoke hearts
- Beans (all kinds, including black beans, garbanzo beans, pinto beans, lentils, black-eyed peas) *Note:* Baked beans tend to be higher in sugar.
- Fish (tuna, salmon, sardines)
- Fruits (canned in natural juice, not syrup)

- Olives
- Roasted red peppers
- Soups and broths (low sodium)
- Tomatoes (no added sugar)
- Water chestnuts

Cereals
- Cold (at least 4 grams of fiber per serving; sugar not listed as one of first two ingredients)
- Hot (at least 4 grams of fiber per serving; e.g., steel-cut oats)

Crackers (at least 3 grams of fiber per serving; zero trans fats)

Herbs and Spices (also see page 227)
- Basil
- Black pepper
- Cardamom
- Cayenne pepper
- Chili pepper
- Cilantro
- Cinnamon
- Cloves
- Coriander
- Cumin
- Curry powder
- Garlic powder
- Ginger
- Nutmeg
- Onion powder
- Oregano
- Paprika
- Parsley
- Rosemary
- Sage

- Sea salt
- Tarragon
- Thyme
- Turmeric
- Vanilla extract

Whole Grains
- Amaranth
- Barley
- Bulgur
- Kasha
- Millet
- Pasta (dry, not canned)
- Quinoa
- Rice (brown, basmati, or wild)
- Wheat berries

Nuts and Seeds
- Almonds
- Cashews
- Peanuts
- Pecans
- Pine nuts
- Pistachios
- Pumpkin seeds
- Sesame seeds
- Sunflower seeds
- Walnuts

Oils
- Canola oil
- Extra virgin olive oil
- High-oleic safflower oil
- Sesame oil (plain or toasted)

Sauces
- Hot sauce
- Pasta sauce
- Soy sauce
- Worcestershire

Vinegars
- Balsamic
- Red wine
- Rice

In the Breadbox

- Whole grain bread ("stone-ground" or "flourless" varieties best)
- Tortillas (at least 3 grams of fiber per serving; will keep longer in the fridge)

Food Group	Glycemic Load[1,2]		
	Low	**Moderate**[3]	**High**
Vegetables	Alfalfa sprouts	Acorn squash	Corn
	Artichoke	Beets	French fries
	Asparagus	Butternut squash	Potato
	Avocado	Green peas	Potato chips
	Bamboo shoots	Parsnips	
	Bean sprouts	Plantain	
	Bok choy	Pumpkin	
	Broccoli	Sweet potato	
	Brussels sprouts	Yam	
	Cabbage		
	Carrots		
	Cauliflower		
	Celery		
	Chard		
	Collard greens		
	Cucumber		
	Eggplant		
	Green beans		
	Kale		
	Kohlrabi		
	Leeks		
	Lettuce		
	Mushrooms		
	Mustard greens		
	Okra		
	Onion		
	Peppers		
	Radish		
	Rutabaga		
	Scallion		
	Snow peas		
	Spinach		
	Summer squash		
	Swiss chard		
	Tomatoes		
	Turnip		
	Water chestnuts		
	Zucchini		

Food Group	Glycemic Load[1,2]		
	Low	**Moderate**[3]	**High**
Fruits	Apples	Apple sauce	Fruit juices and drinks
	Apricot	Banana	
	Berries	Canned fruit	
	Cantaloupe	Dried fruit	
	Cherries	Mango	
	Clementines	Papaya	
	Grapefruit	Pineapple	
	Grapes	Watermelon	
	Honeydew		
	Kiwi		
	Lemon		
	Lime		
	Nectarines		
	Oranges		
	Peaches		
	Pears		
	Plums		
	Tangelos		
	Tangerines		
Legumes	Beans (all kinds except baked)	Baked beans	
	Chickpeas		
	Hummus		
	Lentils		
	Split peas		
	Black-eyed peas		
Nuts	Almonds	Peanut butter, sugar-sweetened	
	Cashews		
	Peanut butter, no added sugar		
	Peanuts		
	Pecans		
	Pistachios		
	Walnuts		

Food Group	Glycemic Load[1,2]		
	Low	Moderate[3]	High
Dairy	Cheese Milk Yogurt, no added sugar		
Grains		Amaranth Barley Bread, minimally processed (including whole kernel, sprouted grain, and stone ground) Breakfast cereal, high fiber Brown rice (varies by type) Bulgur Kasha Millet Pasta (not canned) Quinoa Wheat berries Wild rice	Bread, highly processed (including, bagel, buns, cornbread, English muffin, pita, rolls, and white bread) Breakfast cereals, low fiber Couscous Crackers Pancakes\ Pasta (canned) Pizza Popcorn Pretzels Rice cakes Stuffing Taco shell Tortilla Waffles White rice

[1]For a comprehensive numerical listing of glycemic index and glycemic load, see http://www.glycemicindex.com/.
[2]Most sugary desserts and soft drinks have a high glycemic load.
[3]To help distinguish between related foods (starchy and nonstarchy vegetables, for example), the numerical range for glycemic load categories varies somewhat by food group.

RECOMMENDED READING

Childhood Obesity

Jukes, Mavis, and Lilian Wai-Lin Cheung. *Be Healthy! It's a Girl Thing: Food, Fitness, and Feeling Great.* New York: Random House, 2003.

Kaufman, Francine R. *Diabesity: The Obesity-Diabetes Epidemic That Threatens America — and What We Must Do to Stop It.* New York: Random House, 2005.

Okie, Susan. *Fed up! Winning the War Against Childhood Obesity.* Washington, D.C.: Joseph Henry Press, 2005.

Sothern, Melinda, Heidi Schumacher, and T. Kristian Von Allman. *Trim Kids: The Proven 12-Week Plan That Has Helped Thousands of Children Achieve a Healthier Weight.* New York: HarperCollins, 2001.

Diet and Cookbooks

Agatston, Arthur. *The South Beach Diet.* New York: Rodale Books, 2003.

Brand-Miller, Jennie, Kaye Foster-Powell, and Johanna Burani. *The Low GI Diet Revolution: The Definitive Science-Based Weight Loss Plan.* New York: Marlowe, 2005.

Hyman, Mark. *Ultrametabolism: The Simple Plan for Automatic Weight Loss.* New York: Simon & Schuster, 2006.

Katzen, Mollie. *New Moosewood Cookbook*. Berkeley, Calif.: Ten Speed Press, 2000.

Katzen, Mollie, and Walter Willett. *Eat, Drink, and Weigh Less: A Flexible and Delicious Way to Shrink Your Waist Without Going Hungry*. New York: Hyperion, 2006.

Rolls, Barbara. *Volumetrics Eating Plan*. New York: HarperCollins, 2005.

Sears, Barry. *The Zone: A Dietary Road Map*. New York: HarperCollins, 1995.

Woodruff, Sandra. *Good Carb Cookbook: Secrets of Eating Low on the Glycemic Index*. New York: Avery, 2001.

Politics, Ethics, and Environment

Brownell, Kelly, and Katherine Battle Horgen. *Food Fight: The Inside Story of the Food Industry, America's Obesity Crisis, and What We Can Do About It*. New York: McGraw-Hill, 2004.

Critser, Greg. *Fat Land: How Americans Became the Fattest People in the World*. New York: Houghton Mifflin, 2004.

Jacobson, Michael F. *Six Arguments for a Greener Diet: How a Plant-Based Diet Could Save Your Health and the Environment*. Washington, D.C.: Center for Science in the Public Interest, 2006.

Kimbrell, Andrew, ed. *The Fatal Harvest Reader: The Tragedy of Industrial Agriculture*. Sausalito, Calif.: Foundation for Deep Ecology, 2002.

Linn, Susan. *Consuming Kids: The Hostile Takeover of Childhood*. New York: The New Press, 2004.

Nestle, Marion. *Food Politics: How the Food Industry Influences Nutrition and Health*. Berkeley: University of California Press, 2003.

Pollan, Michael. *The Omnivore's Dilemma: A Natural History of Four Meals*. New York: Penguin Press, 2006.

Schlosser, Eric. *Fast Food Nation: The Dark Side of the All-American Meal*. New York: Houghton Mifflin, 2001.

Spurlock, Morgan. *Don't Eat This Book*. New York: Penguin Group, 2005.

Psychology and Spirituality

Albers, Susan. *Eating Mindfully: How to End Mindless Eating and Enjoy a Balanced Relationship with Food*. Oakland, Calif.: New Harbinger Publications, 2003.

Rimm, Sylvia, and Eric Rimm. *Rescuing the Emotional Lives of Overweight Children*. New York: Rodale Books, 2005.

Schatz, Hale Sophia, and Shira Shaiman. *If the Buddha Came to Dinner: How to Nourish Your Body to Awaken Your Spirit*. New York: Hyperion, 2004.

Thich Nhat Hanh. *Peace Is Every Step: The Path of Mindfulness in Everyday Life*. New York: Bantam Books, 1992.

NOTES

1. Overweight and Overpowered

Page

9 *The percentage of overweight children:* See Strauss, R. S., and Pollack, H. A., "Epidemic increase in childhood overweight, 1986–1998," *JAMA* 2001, 286:2845–2848. Also Ogden, C. L., Carroll, M. D., Curtin L. R., et al., "Prevalence of overweight and obesity in the United States, 1999–2004," *JAMA* 2006, 295:1549–1555.

10 *Pediatricians now regularly diagnose:* See Ebbeling, C. B., Pawlak, D. B., and Ludwig, D. S., "Childhood obesity: public health crisis, common sense cure," *Lancet* 2002, 360:473–482.

One study found that when fifth: See Latner, J. D., and Stunkard, A. J., "Getting worse: the stigmatization of obese children," *Obes Res* 2003, 11:452–456.

Other research shows that being very overweight: See Schwimmer, J. B., Burwinkle, T. M., and Varni, J. W., "Health-related quality of life of severely obese children and adolescents," *JAMA* 2003, 289:1813–1819.

Studies show that when overweight adolescents: See Gortmaker, S. L., Must, A., Perrin, J. M., Sobol, A. M., and Dietz, W. H., "Social and economic consequences of overweight in adolescence and young adulthood," *N Engl J Med* 1993, 329:1008–1012.

11 *Children who develop type 2 diabetes:* See Dean, H., and Flett, B., "Natural history of type 2 diabetes diagnosed in childhood: long-term follow-up in young adult years," *Diabetes* 2002, 51:A24 (abstract). Also Ludwig, D. S., and Ebbeling, C. B., "Type 2 diabetes in children: primary care and public health considerations," *JAMA* 2001, 286:1427–1430.

11 *Shockingly, overweight adolescent girls:* See van Dam, R. M., Willett, W. C., Manson, J. E., and Hu, F. B., "The relationship between overweight in adolescence and premature death in women," *Annals Int Med* 2006, 145:91–97.

And according to a study we did: See Olshansky, S. J., Passaro, D. J., Hershow, R. C., et al., "A potential decline in life expectancy in the United States in the 21st century," *N Engl J Med* 2005, 352:1138–1145.

Some scientists have proposed: See Speakman, J. R., "Thrifty genes for obesity and the metabolic syndrome — time to call off the search?" *Diab Vasc Dis Res* 2006, 3:7–11.

12 *The second problem:* See Leibel, R. L., Rosenbaum, M., and Hirsch, J., "Changes in energy expenditure resulting from altered body weight," *N Engl J Med* 1995, 332:621–628.

Research from our laboratory: See Agus, M. S. D., Swain, J. F., Larson, C. L., Eckert, E. A., and Ludwig, D. S., "Dietary composition and the physiologic adaptations to energy restriction," *Am J Clin Nutr* 2000, 71:901–907. Also Ludwig, D. S., "The glycemic index: physiological mechanisms relating to obesity, diabetes and cardiovascular disease," *JAMA* 2002, 287:2414–2423. Also Pereira, M. A., Swain, J., Goldfine, A. B., Rifai, N., and Ludwig, D. S., "Effects of a low glycemic load diet on resting energy expenditure and heart disease risk factors during weight loss," *JAMA* 2004, 292: 2482–2490.

13 *What has changed:* See Wadden, T. A., Brownell, K. D., and Foster, G. D., "Obesity: responding to the global epidemic," *J Consult Clin Psychol* 2002, 70:510–525. Also Brownell, K., and Horgen, K. B., *Food Fight: The Inside Story of the Food Industry, America's Obesity Crisis, and What We Can Do About It* (New York: McGraw-Hill, 2004).

15 *Biologically, humans are born:* See Benton, D., "Role of parents in the determination of the food preferences of children and the development of obesity," *Int J Obes Relat Metab Disord* 2004, 28:858–869.

16 *Research shows that young children:* See Rolls, B. J., Engell, D., and Birch, L. L., "Serving portion size influences 5-year-old but not 3-year-old children's food intake," *J Am Diet Assoc* 2000, 100:232–234.

Supersizing may actually erode: See Ebbeling, C. B., Sinclair, K. B., Pereira, M. A., Garcia-Lago, E., Feldman, H. A., and Ludwig, D. S., "Compensation for energy intake from fast food among overweight and lean adolescents," *JAMA* 2004, 291:2828–2833.

2. Welcoming Children to Weight Loss: A Day at the OWL Clinic

20 *A Day at the OWL Clinic:* These three articles discuss the evaluation and management of childhood obesity and its complications. See Ludwig, D. S., and Ebbeling, C. B., "Type 2 diabetes in children: primary care and public health considerations," *JAMA* 2001, 286:1427–1430. Also Ebbeling, C. B., Pawlak, D. B., and Ludwig, D. S., "Childhood obesity: public health crisis, common sense cure," *Lan-*

cet 2002, 360:473–482. Also Dietz, W. H., and Robinson, T. N., "Clinical practice: overweight children and adolescents," *N Engl J Med* 2005, 352:2100–2109.

32 *Can You "Catch" Obesity?:* See Henig, R. M., "Fat Factors," *New York Times Magazine,* August 13, 2006.

3. Eating to Feel Full

46 *The command center:* See Lustig, R. H., "The neuroendocrinology of childhood obesity," *Pediatr Clin North Am* 2001, 48:909–930.

49 *All carbohydrates are composed:* These three review articles examine how high–glycemic index carbohydrate affects health, a topic considered throughout this chapter. See Ludwig, D. S., "Dietary glycemic index and obesity," *J Nutr* 2000, 130:280S–283S. Also Ludwig, D. S., "The glycemic index: physiological mechanisms relating to obesity, diabetes and cardiovascular disease," *JAMA* 2002, 287:2414–2423. Also Ludwig, D. S., "Glycemic load comes of age," *J Nutr* 2003, 133:2695–2696.

50 *Jenkins unveiled this:* See Jenkins, D. J., Wolever, T. M., Taylor, R. H., et al., "Glycemic index of foods: a physiological basis for carbohydrate exchange," *Am J Clin Nutr* 1981, 34:362–366.

51 *In 1997, Walter Willett:* See Salmeron, J., Manson, J. E., Stampfer, M. J., Colditz, G. A., Wing, A. L., and Willett, W. C., "Dietary fiber, glycemic load, and risk of non-insulin-dependent diabetes mellitus in women," *JAMA* 1997, 277:472–477.

We decided to test: See Ludwig, D. S., Majzoub, J. A., Al-Zahrani, A., Dallal, G. E., Blanco, I., and Roberts, S. B., "High glycemic index foods, overeating, and obesity," *Pediatrics* 1999, 103:E26.

53 *In a classic experiment:* See Thompson, D. A., and Campbell, R. G., "Hunger in humans induced by 2-deoxy-D-glucose: glucoprivic control of taste preference and food intake," *Science* 1977, 198:1065–1068.

More than a dozen: See Ludwig, D. S., "Dietary glycemic index and obesity," *J Nutr* 2000, 130:280S–283S. Also Ball, S. D., Keller, K. R., Moyer-Mileur, L. J., Ding, Y. W., Donaldson, D., and Jackson, W. D., "Prolongation of satiety after low versus moderately high glycemic index meals in obese adolescents," *Pediatrics* 2003, 111:488–494. Also Warren, J. M., Henry, C. J., and Simonite, V., "Low glycemic index breakfasts and reduced food intake in preadolescent children," *Pediatrics* 2003, 112:E414.

54 *One explanation:* See Leibel, R. L., Rosenbaum, M., and Hirsch, J., "Changes in energy expenditure resulting from altered body weight," *N Engl J Med* 1995, 332:621–628.

To find out if low-glycemic: See Pereira, M. A., Swain, J., Goldfine, A. B., Rifai, N., and Ludwig, D. S., "Effects of a low–glycemic load diet on resting energy expenditure and heart disease risk factors during weight loss," *JAMA* 2004, 292:2482–2490.

We have extended: See Spieth, L. E., Harnish, J. D., Lenders, C. M., et al., "A low–glycemic index diet in the treatment of pediatric obesity," *Arch Pediatr Adolesc Med* 2000, 154:947–951. Also Ebbeling, C. B., Leidig, M. M., Sinclair, K. B., Hangen, J. P., and Ludwig, D. S., "A reduced–glycemic load diet in the treatment of adolescent obesity," *Arch Pediatr Adolesc Med* 2003, 157:773–779. Also Ebbeling, C. B., Leidig, M. M., Sinclair, K. B., Seger-Shippee, L. G., Feldman, H. A., and Ludwig, D. S., "Effects of an ad libitum low–glycemic load diet on cardiovascular disease risk factors in obese young adults," *Am J Clin Nutr* 2005, 81:976–982.

55 *Based on these and other:* See Slabber, M., Barnard, H. C., Kuyl, J. M., Dannhauser, A., and Schall, R., "Effects of a low-insulin-response, energy-restricted diet on weight loss and plasma insulin concentrations in hyperinsulinemic obese females," *Am J Clin Nutr* 1994, 60:48–53. Also Clapp, J. I., "Diet, exercise, and feto-placental growth," *Arch Gynecol Obstet* 1997, 261:101–107. Also Dumesnil, J. G., Turgeon, J., Tremblay, A., et al., "Effect of a low-glycaemic index-low-fat-high-protein diet on the atherogenic metabolic risk profile of abdominally obese men," *Br J Nutr* 2001, 86:557–568. Also Bouché, C., Rizkalla, S. W., Luo, J., et al., "Five-week, low–glycemic index diet decreases total fat mass and improves plasma lipid profile in moderately overweight nondiabetic men," *Diabetes Care* 2002, 25:822–828. Also McMillan-Price, J., Petocz, P., Atkinson, F., et al., "Comparison of 4 diets of varying glycemic load on weight loss and cardiovascular risk reduction in overweight and obese young adults: a randomized controlled trial," *Arch Intern Med* 2006, 166:1466–1475.

We set out to answer: See Pawlak, D. B., Kushner, J. A., and Ludwig, D. S., "Effects of dietary glycaemic index on adiposity, glucose homeostasis, and plasma lipids in animals," *Lancet* 2004, 364:778–785.

59 *The link between high-glycemic:* See Salmeron, J., Manson, J. E., Stampfer, M. J., Colditz, G. A., Wing, A. L., and Willett, W. C., "Dietary fiber, glycemic load, and risk of non-insulin-dependent diabetes mellitus in women," *JAMA* 1997, 277:472–477. Also Liu, S., Willett, W. C., Stampfer, M. J., et al., "A prospective study of dietary glycemic load, carbohydrate intake, and risk of coronary heart disease in U.S. women," *Am J Clin Nutr* 2000, 71:1455–1461. Also Ludwig, D. S., "Glycemic load comes of age," *J Nutr* 2003, 133:2695–2696. Also Oh, K., Hu, F. B., Cho, E., et al., "Carbohydrate intake, glycemic index, glycemic load, and dietary fiber in relation to risk of stroke in women," *Am J Epidemiol* 2005, 161:161–169. Also Ma, Y., Olendzki, B., Chiriboga, D., et al., "Association between dietary carbohydrates and body weight," *Am J Epidemiol* 2005, 161:359–367.

High-glycemic foods may also: See Biddinger, S. B., and Ludwig, D. S., "The insulin-like growth factor axis: a potential link between glycemic index and cancer," *Am J Clin Nutr* 2005, 82:277–278. Also Ludwig, D. S., "Glycemic load comes of age," *J Nutr* 2003, 133:2695–2696.

60 *David Benton at the University of Wales:* See Benton, D., Ruffin, M. P., Lassel, T., et al., "The delivery rate of dietary carbohydrates affects cognitive performance in both rats and humans," *Psychopharmacology* (Berl) 2003, 166:86–90.

In a study from Toronto: See Papanikolaou, Y., Palmer, H., Binns, M. A.,

Jenkins, D. J., and Greenwood, C. E., "Better cognitive performance following a low-glycaemic-index compared with a high-glycaemic-index carbohydrate meal in adults with type 2 diabetes," *Diabetologia* 2006, 49:855–862.

61 *For this reason, we examined:* See Pereira, M. A., Kartashov, A. I., Ebbeling, C. B., et al., "Fast-food habits, weight gain, and insulin resistance (the CARDIA study): 15-year prospective analysis," *Lancet* 2005, 365:36–42.

63 *Among apparently healthy Italians:* See Valtueña, S., Pellegrini, N., Ardigò, D., et al., "Dietary glycemic index and liver steatosis," *Am J Clin Nutr* 2006, 84:136–142.

In fact, research from our laboratory: See Ludwig, D. S., Pereira, M. A., Kroenke, C. H., et al., "Dietary fiber, weight gain and cardiovascular disease risk factors in young adults: the CARDIA study," *JAMA* 1999, 282:1539–1546. Also Pirozzo, S., Summerbell, C., Cameron, C., and Glasziou, P., "Should we recommend low-fat diets for obesity?" *Obes Rev* 2003, 4:83–90.

These diets do produce: See Foster, G. D., Wyatt, H. R., Hill, J. O., et al., "A randomized trial of a low-carbohydrate diet for obesity," *N Engl J Med* 2003, 348:2082–2090.

64 *Among women in the Nurses' Health Study:* See Chiu, C. J., Hubbard, L. D., Armstrong, J., et al., "Dietary glycemic index and carbohydrate in relation to early age-related macular degeneration," *Am J Clin Nutr* 2006, 83:880–886.

65 *In addition, they usually:* See Ledikwe, J. H., Blanck, H. M., Kettel, K. L., et al., "Dietary energy density is associated with energy intake and weight status in U.S. adults," *Am J Clin Nutr* 2006, 83:1362–1368. Also Bell, E. A., and Rolls, B. J., "Energy density of foods affects energy intake across multiple levels of fat content in lean and obese women," *Am J Clin Nutr* 2001, 73:1010–1018.

66 *Can eating too much:* See Liu, S., Manson, J. E., Stampfer, M. J., et al., "A prospective study of whole-grain intake and risk of type 2 diabetes mellitus in U.S. women," *Am J Public Health* 2000, 90:1409–1415. Also Hu, F. B., and Willett, W. C., "Optimal diets for prevention of coronary heart disease," *JAMA* 2002, 288:2569–2578. Also Steffen, L. M., Jacobs, D. R., Jr., Stevens, J., Shahar, E., Carithers, T., and Folsom, A. R., "Associations of whole-grain, refined-grain, and fruit and vegetable consumption with risks of all-cause mortality and incident coronary artery disease and ischemic stroke: the Atherosclerosis Risk in Communities (ARIC) Study," *Am J Clin Nutr* 2003, 78:383–390.

67 *The fact is:* See Jacobson, M. F., *Six Arguments for a Greener Diet: How a Plant-Based Diet Could Save Your Health and the Environment* (Washington, D.C.: Center for Science in the Public Interest, 2006).

69 *According to one Australian study:* See Smith, R., Mann, N., Braue, A., and Varigos, G., "Low glycemic load, high protein diet lessens facial acne severity," *Asia Pac J Clin Nutr* 2005, 14(Suppl):S97.

Whereas unsaturated fats: See Kavanagh, K., Jones, K., Sawyer, J., Kelly, K., Wagner, J. D., and Rudel, L. L., "Trans fat diet induces insulin resistance in monkeys," *American Diabetes Association* 2006 (abstract).

71 *However, high–glycemic index foods:* See Bornet, F. R., Costagliola, D., Rizkalla, S. W., et al., "Insulinemic and glycemic indexes of six starch-rich foods taken alone and in mixed meal by type 2 diabetics," *Am J Clin Nutr* 1987, 45:588–595. Also Chew, I., Brand, J. C., Thorburn, A. W., and Truswell, A. S., "Application of glycemic index to mixed meals," *Am J Clin Nutr* 1988, 47:53–56. Also Wolever, T. M., and Bolognesi, C., "Prediction of glucose and insulin responses of normal subjects after consuming mixed meals varying in energy, protein, fat, carbohydrate and glycemic index," *J Nutr* 1996 126:2807–2812.

71 *Instead, as Marion Nestle:* See Nestle, M., *Food Politics: How the Food Industry Influences Nutrition and Health* (Berkeley: University of California Press, 2003).

72 *In one study, investigators:* See Levin, B. E., and Govek, E., "Gestational obesity accentuates obesity in obesity-prone progeny," *Am J Physiol* 1998, 275:R1374–R1379.

Recently published research suggests: See Moses, R. G., Luebcke, M., Davis, W. S., et al., "The effect of a low glycemic index diet during pregnancy on obstetric outcomes," *Am J Clin Nutr* 2006, 84:807–812.

Regarding factors in infancy: See Harder, T., Bergmann, R., Kallischnigg, G., and Plagemann, A., "Duration of breastfeeding and risk of overweight: a meta-analysis," *Am J Epidemiol* 2005, 162:397–403.

4. Getting Physical

75 *According to a Kaiser:* See Henry J. Kaiser Family Foundation, "Generation M: media in the lives of 8–18 year olds," 2005, http://www.kff.org/entmedia/entmedia030905pkg.cfm.

Amazingly, ten- to sixteen-year-olds: See Strauss, R. S., Rodzilsky, D., Burack, G., et al., "Psychosocial correlates of physical activity in healthy children," *Arch Pediatr Adolesc Med* 2001, 155:897–902.

77 *And as shown by Robert Whitaker:* See Burdette, H. L., and Whitaker, R. C., "Resurrecting free play in young children: looking beyond fitness and fatness to attention, affiliation, and affect," *Arch Pediatr Adolesc Med* 2005, 159:46–50.

78 *To illustrate this point:* See Levine, J. A., Lanningham-Foster, L. M., McCrady, S. K., et al., "Interindividual variation in posture allocation: possible role in human obesity," *Science* 2005, 307:584–586.

79 *To examine this point:* See Pawlak, D. B., Kushner, J. A., and Ludwig, D. S., "Effects of dietary glycaemic index on adiposity, glucose homeostasis, and plasma lipids in animals," *Lancet* 2004, 364:778–785.

80 *As described in chapter 3:* See Pereira, M. A., Swain, J., Goldfine, A. B., Rifai, N., and Ludwig, D. S., "Effects of a low–glycemic load diet on resting energy expenditure and heart disease risk factors during weight loss," *JAMA* 2004, 292:2482–2490.

When researchers gave: See DeMarco, H. M., Sucher, K. P., Cisar, C. J., and

Butterfield, G. E., "Pre-exercise carbohydrate meals: application of glycemic index," *Med Sci Sports Exerc* 1999, 31:164–170.

81 *Among 20,000 adolescent:* See De Moor, M. H., Beem, A. L., Stubbe, J. H., Boomsma, D. I., and De Geus, E. J., "Regular exercise, anxiety, depression and personality: a population-based study," *Prev Med* 2006, 42:273–279.

In England, nine- and ten-year-old: See Williamson, D., Dewey, A., and Steinberg, H., "Mood change through physical exercise in nine- to ten-year-old children," *Percept Mot Skills* 2001, 93:311–316.

And researchers in Japan: See Nabkasorn, C., Miyai, N., Sootmongkol, A., et al., "Effects of physical exercise on depression, neuroendocrine stress hormones and physiological fitness in adolescent females with depressive symptoms," *Eur J Public Health* 2006, 16:179–184.

84 *In one study involving:* See von Kries, R., Toschke, A. M., Wurmser, H., Sauerwald, T., and Koletzko, B., "Reduced risk for overweight and obesity in 5- and 6-y-old children by duration of sleep — a cross-sectional study," *Int J Obes Relat Metab Disord* 2002, 26:710–716.

85 *In a landmark study:* See Gortmaker, S. L., Must, A., Sobol, A. M., Peterson, K., Colditz, G. A., and Dietz, W. H., "Television viewing as a cause of increasing obesity among children in the United States, 1986–1990," *Arch Pediatr Adolesc Med* 1996, 150:356–362.

A similar conclusion: See Lumeng, J. C., Rahnama, S., Appugliese, D., Kaciroti, N., and Bradley, R. H., "Television exposure and overweight risk in preschoolers," *Arch Pediatr Adolesc Med* 2006, 160:417–422.

And in a third study: See Kaur, H., Choi, W. S., Mayo, M. S., and Harris, K. J., "Duration of television watching is associated with increased body mass index," *J Pediatr* 2003, 143:506–511.

86 *Robert Klesges and colleagues:* See Klesges, R. C., Shelton, M. L., and Klesges, L. M., "Effects of television on metabolic rate: potential implications for childhood obesity," *Pediatrics* 1993, 91:281–286.

87 *Epstein's team performed:* See Epstein, L. H., Paluch, R. A., Consalvi, A., Riordan, K., and Scholl, T., "Effects of manipulating sedentary behavior on physical activity and food intake," *J Pediatr* 2002, 140:334–339.

Tom Robinson at Stanford: See Robinson, T. N., "Reducing children's television viewing to prevent obesity: a randomized controlled trial," *JAMA* 1999, 282:1561–1567.

Leann Birch at Penn State: See Francis, L. A., and Birch, L. L., "Does eating during television viewing affect preschool children's intake?" *J Am Diet Assoc* 2006, 106:598–600.

88 *Studies clearly show:* See Borzekowski, D. L., and Robinson, T. N., "The 30-second effect: an experiment revealing the impact of television commercials on food preferences of preschoolers," *J Am Diet Assoc* 2001, 101:42–46. Also Coon, K. A., and Tucker, K. L., "Television and children's consumption patterns: a review of the literature," *Minerva Pediatr* 2002, 54:423–436. Also Ludwig, D. S., and

Gortmaker, S. L., "Programming obesity in childhood," *Lancet* 2004, 364:226–227. Also Henry J. Kaiser Family Foundation, "The role of media in childhood obesity," 2004, http://www.kff.org/entmedia/entmedia022404pkg.cfm. Also Institute of Medicine, *Food Marketing to Children and Youth: Threat or Opportunity?*" ed. J. M. McGinnis (Washington, D.C.: National Academies Press, 2006).

89 *In her powerful book:* See Nestle, M., *Food Politics: How the Food Industry Influences Nutrition and Health* (Berkeley: University of California Press, 2003).

A recent study by Steven Gortmaker: See also Wiecha, J. L., Peterson, K. E., Ludwig, D. S., Kim, J., Sobol, A., and Gortmaker, S. L., "When children eat what they watch: impact of television viewing on dietary intake in youth," *Arch Pediatr Adolesc Med* 2006, 160:436–442.

Researchers in New Zealand: See Hancox, R. J., Milne, B. J., and Poulton, R., "Association between child and adolescent television viewing and adult health: a longitudinal birth cohort study," *Lancet* 2004, 364:257–262.

90 *Fifty-nine overweight:* See Carrel, A. L., Clark, R. R., Peterson, S. E., Nemeth, B. A., Sullivan, J., and Allen, D. B., "Improvement of fitness, body composition, and insulin sensitivity in overweight children in a school-based exercise program: a randomized, controlled study," *Arch Pediatr Adolesc Med* 2005, 159:963–968.

These conditions don't: See Young-Hyman, D., Schlundt, D. G., Herman, L., DeLuca, F., and Counts, D., "Evaluation of the insulin resistance syndrome in 5- to 10-year-old overweight/obese African-American children," *Diabetes Care* 2001, 24:1359–1364.

A study of overweight children: See Kelly, A. S., Wetzsteon, R. J., Kaiser, D. R., et al., "Inflammation, insulin, and endothelial function in overweight children and adolescents: the role of exercise," *J Pediatr* 2004, 145:731–736.

Among a group of Caucasian girls: See Valdimarsson, O., Sigurdsson, G., Steingrimsdottir, L., and Karlsson, M. K., "Physical activity in the post-pubertal period is associated with maintenance of pre-pubertal high bone density — a 5-year follow-up," *Scand J Med Sci Sports* 2005, 15:280–286.

91 *Consider the findings:* See Kimm, S. Y., Glynn, N. W., Kriska, A. M., et al., "Longitudinal changes in physical activity in a biracial cohort during adolescence," *Med Sci Sports Exerc* 2000, 32:1445–1454.

As summarized by William Dietz: See Dietz, W. H., "You are what you eat — what you eat is what you are," *J Adolesc Health Care* 1990, 11:76–81.

94 *To demonstrate this point:* See Maffeis, C., Zaffanello, M., Pellegrino, M., et al., "Nutrient oxidation during moderately intense exercise in obese prepubertal boys," *J Clin Endocrinol Metab* 2005, 90:231–236.

97 *For example, researchers in France:* See Wagner, A., Klein-Platat, C., Arveiler, D., Haan, M. C., Schlienger, J. L., and Simon, C., "Parent-child physical activity relationships in 12-year-old French students do not depend on family socioeconomic status," *Diabetes Metab* 2004, 30:359–366.

5. It's the Thought That Counts

100 *In one study, researchers:* See Morrison, T. G., Kalin, R., and Morrison, M. A., "Body-image evaluation and body-image investment among adolescents: a test of sociocultural and social comparison theories," *Adolescence* 2004, 39:571–592.

103 *In one study, researchers found:* See Kenardy, J., Arnow, B., and Agras, W. S., "The aversiveness of specific emotional states associated with binge-eating in obese subjects," *Austr N Z J Psychiatry* 1996, 30:839–844. For a review article on the topic, see Heatherton, T. F., and Baumeister, R. F., "Binge eating as escape from self-awareness," *Psychol Bull* 1991, 110:86–108.

106 *In 1997, I conducted:* See Ludwig, D. S., Majzoub, J. A., Al-Zahrani, A., Dallal, G. E., Blanco, I., and Roberts, S. B., "High glycemic index foods, overeating, and obesity," *Pediatrics* 1999, 103:E26.

108 *The tendency to eat:* See Wansink, B., Painter, J. E., and Lee, Y. K., "The office candy dish: proximity's influence on estimated and actual consumption," *Int J Obes* 2006, 30:871–875.

110 *Researchers in Finland:* See Marniemi, J., Kronholm, E., Aunola, S., et al., "Visceral fat and psychosocial stress in identical twins discordant for obesity," *J Intern Med* 2002, 251:35–43.

115 *Consider another study:* See Wansink, B., Painter, J. E., and North, J., "Bottomless bowls: why visual cues of portion size may influence intake," *Obes Res* 2005, 13:93–100.

116 *So they studied a group:* See Hallberg, L., Bjorn-Rasmussen, E., Rossander, L., and Suwanik, R., "Iron absorption from Southeast Asian diets. II. Role of various factors that might explain low absorption," *Am J Clin Nutr* 1977, 30:539–548.

6. There's No Place Like Home

125 *Children are born:* See Benton, D., "Role of parents in the determination of the food preferences of children and the development of obesity," *Int J Obes Relat Metab Disord* 2004, 28:858–869.

Leann Birch at Pennsylvania State: See Addessi, E., Galloway, A. T., Visalberghi, E., and Birch, L. L., "Specific social influences on the acceptance of novel foods in 2–5-year-old children," *Appetite* 2005, 45:264–271.

126 *Other research by Birch:* See Birch, L. L., Gunder, L., Grimm-Thomas, K., and Laing, D. G., "Infants' consumption of a new food enhances acceptance of similar foods," *Appetite* 1998, 30:283–295.

127 *When it comes to body weight:* See Golan, M., Weizman, A., Apter, A., and Fainaru, M., "Parents as the exclusive agents of change in the treatment of childhood obesity," *Am J Clin Nutr* 1998, 67:1130–1135.

129 *Leonard Epstein:* See Wrotniak, B. H., Epstein, L. H., Paluch, R. A., and Roemmich, J. N., "Parent weight change as a predictor of child weight change in

family-based behavioral obesity treatment," *Arch Pediatr Adolesc Med* 2004, 158:342–347.

129 *Another study by Epstein's:* See Stein, R. I., Epstein, L. H., Raynor, H. A., Kilanowski, C. K., and Paluch, R. A., "The influence of parenting change on pediatric weight control," *Obes Res* 2005, 13:1749–1755.

Tweens' increasing reasoning: For a comprehensive, scholarly consideration of many parenting issues considered in this chapter, see Bornstein, M., ed., *Handbook of Parenting,* 2nd ed., vol. 1 (London: Lawrence Erlbaum Associates, 2002).

131 *Mary Story:* See Boutelle, K. N., Lytle, L. A., Murray, D. M., Birnbaum, A. S., and Story, M., "Perceptions of the family mealtime environment and adolescent mealtime behavior: do adults and adolescents agree?" *J Nutr Ed* 2001, 33:128–133.

132 *In a striking illustration:* See Fulkerson, J. A., McGuire, M. T., Neumark-Sztainer, D., Story, M., French, S. A., and Perry, C. L., "Weight-related attitudes and behaviors of adolescent boys and girls who are encouraged to diet by their mothers," *Int J Obes Relat Metab Disord* 2002, 26:1579–1587.

133 *And according to recent data:* See Rhee, K. W., Lumeng, J. C., Appugliese, D. P., Kaciroti, N., and Bradley, R. H., "Parenting styles and overweight status in first grade," *Pediatrics* 2006, 117:2047–2054.

135 *Leann Birch and colleagues:* See Galloway, A. T., Fiorito, L. M., Francis, L. A., and Birch, L. L., "'Finish your soup': counterproductive effects of pressuring children to eat on intake and affect," *Appetite* 2006, 46:318–323.

Conversely, according to another study: See Birch, L. L., Fisher, J. O., and Davison, K. K., "Learning to overeat: maternal use of restrictive feeding practices promotes girls' eating in the absence of hunger," *Am J Clin Nutr* 2003, 78:215–220.

137 *To illustrate this point:* See Newman, J., and Taylor, A., "Effect of a means-end contingency on young children's food preferences," *J Exp Child Psychol* 1992, 53:200–216.

139 *Studies by Walter Mischel:* See Mischel, W., Shoda, Y., and Rodriguez, M. L., "Delay of gratification in children," *Science* 1989, 244:933–938.

In fact, a study by Dianne Neumark-Sztainer: See Larson, N. I., Story, M., Eisenberg, M. E., and Neumark-Sztainer, D., "Food preparation and purchasing roles among adolescents: associations with sociodemographic characteristics and diet quality," *J Am Diet Assoc* 2006, 106:211–218.

145 *Research has shown:* See Gillman, M. W., Rifas-Shiman, S. L., Frazier, A. L., et al., "Family dinner and diet quality among older children and adolescents," *Arch Fam Med* 2000, 9:235–240. Also Neumark-Sztainer, D., Hannan, P. J., Story, M., Croll, J., and Perry, C., "Family meal patterns: associations with socio-demographic characteristics and improved dietary intake among adolescents," *J Am Diet Assoc* 2003, 103:317–322. Also Videon, T. M., and Manning, C. K., "Influences on adolescent eating patterns: the importance of family meals," *J Adolesc Health* 2003, 32:365–373.

In addition, they are: See Taveras, E. M., Rifas-Shiman, S. L., Berkey, C. S., et al., "Family dinner and adolescent overweight," *Obes Res* 2005, 13:900–906.

146 *A study by Len Epstein:* See Raynor, H. A., Kilanowski, C. K., Esterlis, I., and Epstein, L. H., "A cost-analysis of adopting a healthful diet in a family-based obesity treatment program," *J Am Diet Assoc* 2002, 102:645–656.

7. The 9-Week Program

173 *Researchers examined the effects:* See Oka, K., Sakuarae, A., Fujise, T., Yoshimatsu, H., Sakata, T., and Nakata, M., "Food texture differences affect energy metabolism in rats," *J Dent Res* 2003, 82:491–494.

In humans, chewing gum: See Levine, J., Baukol, P., and Pavlidis, I., "The energy expended in chewing gum," *N Engl J Med* 1999, 341:2100.

8. Changing The World

193 *For this reason, we examined:* See Lesser, L. I., Ebbeling, C. B., Goozner, M., Wypij, D., and Ludwig, D. S. "Relationship between funding source and conclusion among nutrition-related scientific articles," *PLOS Med* 2007, 4:E5

INDEX